THE STERILIZATION CONTROVERSY

THE STERILIZATION CONTROVERSY

A New Crisis for the Catholic Hospital?

By

JOHN P. BOYLE

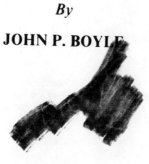

PAULIST PRESS
New York/Ramsey/Toronto

Nihil Obstat
Anthony J. Farrell
Censor Librorum

December 16, 1976

Imprimatur
✠ Gerald O'Keefe
Bishop of Davenport

December 17, 1976

Library of Congress
Catalog Card Number: 77-7378

ISBN: 0-8091-2016-X

Cover Design: Tim McKeen

Published by Paulist Press
Editorial Office: 1865 Broadway, New York, N.Y. 10023
Business Office: 545 Island Road, Ramsey, N.J. 07446

Printed and bound in the
United States of America

Contents

For my parents
Clem A. Boyle
(1895-1965)
and
Marie Phillips Boyle

Abbreviations

AAS   *Acta Apostolicae Sedis*

DB   H. Denzinger and H. Bannwart, *Enchiridion Symbolorum Definitionum et Declarationum de rebus fidei et morum,* 32nd ed. by Karl Rahner, Freiburg: Herder, 1952.

DS   H. Denzinger and A. Schönmetzer, *Enchiridion . . .* Freiburg, 1973.

GS   *Gaudium et Spes* (Pastoral Constitution on the Church in the Modern World).

LG   *Lumen Gentium* (Constitution on the Church).

DH   *Dignitatis Humanae* (Declaration on Religious Freedom).

Neuner-J. Neuner and H. Roos, *The Teaching of the Catholic Roos Church,* ed. by Karl Rahner, trans. by Geoffrey Stevens (Staten Island: Alba House, 1967).

DV   *Dei Verbum* (Constitution on Divine Revelation).

Preface

The problem of sterilization and the Catholic hospital became a concern of mine almost from the beginning of my professional life. Within months of my entrance into university teaching, a nearby Catholic hospital faced the threat of a suit over its sterilization policy. The round of study and consultation that followed soon made it clear to me that many Catholic hospitals were struggling to maintain both their loyalty to the ethical teachings of the Church and their commitment to the health care demanded by their medical staffs and patients. A related loss of their sense of identity by some Catholic hospitals since Vatican II has left them impotent when their very existence has been questioned by health-care planners. A sense of purpose has become a life-and-death matter.

The opportunity to study more systematically the questions raised by the sterilization controversy came from an invitation to lecture at Loras College, Dubuque, in the winter of 1975. The first three chapters of this book grew out of those lectures. A study of the role of the corporation as moral agent came in response to an invitation to participate in a Workshop on Theological Decision-making held in San Francisco in March 1976, under the sponsorship of the National Association of Catholic Chaplains. The fourth chapter emerged from that study. I am grateful both to Loras and the NACC, and they might be grateful if I point out that the opinions in this book are my own.

I dedicate this book to my parents, who have given me life and faith. At crucial moments, the Catholic hospital with the affirmations it represents offered a place for us to ponder the wonder of birth and the mystery of long suffering and death.

School of Religion   John P. Boyle
University of Iowa
Iowa City, Iowa

Introduction

In May 1976,[1] during a debate on sterilization at a London meeting of the European Federation of Catholic Physicians' Associations, Dr. R. G. Thompkins of Tulsa, Oklahoma read the text of a reply on that subject to the National Conference of Catholic Bishops from the Vatican Congregation for the Doctrine of the Faith. The Vatican response repeated modern papal teaching that direct sterilization is an intrinsically evil act.

The NCCB subsequently released the text of the Vatican document, which has an interesting history. For one thing the reply is dated March 13, 1975, and thus had been in the hands of the bishops' conference for more than a year. For another, the response came to questions brought to Rome by the American bishops more than a year before that. The fact that the bishops decided to ask questions of Rome about sterilization at their meeting in November 1973 suggests that the *Code of Ethical and Religious Directives for Catholic Health Facilities* which the bishops had approved overwhelmingly at their 1971 meeting was not being observed: directive 18 of the code forbids direct contraceptive sterilizations.

Yet, despite the fact that the reply had come from Rome in March 1975, and that the substance of the reply had been incorporated on April 14, 1975 into a letter to the bishops from the president of the NCCB, Archbishop Joseph L. Bernardin, the text was not published, and there is little evidence that many bishops took forceful steps to bring Catholic hospitals into compliance with the code. In fact, at their meeting in November 1975, the bishops decided to have a commentary on the document prepared jointly by their committee on doctrine and the USCC committee on health affairs. It was only in December 1975 that the nearly three hundred bishops themselves received the text of the Roman reply. After that it was probably only a matter of time until the text found its way into the public domain. The proposed commentary has not yet appeared.

This brief history of hesitation by the bishops' conference suggests that there is more to the problem of sterilization than first meets the eye. At a time when medical researchers talk seriously about the approach of genetic manipulation in various forms, and genetic screening (with possible abortion following the discovery of a genetic anomaly) is already becoming routine in many cases, it might easily seem quixotic of the bishops and the Vatican to expend energy fulminating against sterilization.

Nevertheless, it seems to me that sterilization is a paradigm of the practical ethical problems faced by Catholic hospitals in the United States, and the argument about it is a paradigm of the differences among bishops and moral theologians in the Church today. The response from the Congregation repeats (predictably, one suspects) the doctrine of the encyclical *Humanae Vitae*, which is itself a restatement of nineteenth- and twentieth-century papal teaching on contraception and sterilization.

The query to Rome was prompted by increasingly widespread practice in Catholic hospitals in the United States and Canada of permitting sterilizations under some circumstances. The rationale for this practice obviously differed from the natural law doctrine of earlier Church statements on sterilization. That doctrine is under widespread attack.

Why did the hospitals permit the sterilizations? That remains a subject for study, but we do know some things. One is that some Catholic hospitals were ordered by courts to permit sterilizations. The hospitals are presently immune to orders of this kind by the federal courts, thanks to an amendment to various bills by Senator Frank Church that prohibits the federal courts from taking jurisdiction on the grounds that the hospitals have received federal money in the form of Hill-Burton or similar grants. Some states too have passed "conscience clauses" that permit institutions to prohibit procedures, like sterilization, to which the hospital has religious or ethical objections. But while the courts have been curbed, other government agencies, especially the newly created health-care facilities planning agencies, exert pressures of their own. There is the constant threat that a hospital which does not provide the "full range of obstetrical services"—including sterilization and abortion—may be refused the "certificate of need" that will permit it to construct or remodel its facilities. Refusal of the certificate of need can mean extinction for the Catholic hospital. Pressures come from insurance carriers and from government programs for various segments of the population, which become a party to the medical treatment of more and more people. The national health insurance so much talked about in the U.S., but not yet in existence, has taken the form of provincial plans in Canada which make Catholic hospitals part of a system of health care delivery under government control.[2]

Catholic hospitals feel other kinds of pressures too. Many of them serve communities or whole areas in which much of the population is not Catholic. In many places, the Catholic hospital is the only readily available health-care facility. The teaching of the Second Vatican Council on religious liberty has had an impact on the hospitals' consideration of the rights of staff physicians and patients who do not share the convictions of the Catholic Church. This respect for the rights of others' conscience is now an important ingredient in a doctrine of cooperation between the hospital, its staff physicians and the public it serves.

Finally, sterilization itself has become easier to perform. Laparoscopic techniques make tubal ligations simpler; vasectomy has become an office procedure. The number of persons choosing to be sterilized has risen sharply. *The New York Times* reported recently that in 1973 seventy percent of American married couples were using some form of contraception, and one-fourth of them had chosen sterilization. The figures are the most recent available and come from the National Center for Health Statistics.[3] Increasing acceptance of sterilization as a contraceptive technique by large segments of the population puts pressure on physicians and on hospitals, particularly at a time of rising consumer militancy in the health-care field.

The sterilization issue is thus paradigmatic of others faced by Catholic hospitals in the United States. Abortion poses many similar problems in the wake of Supreme Court decisions striking down most attempts to restrict the practice. The issues raised by sterilization in one way or other have implications for problems like rights of privacy, euthanasia and many others too.

In this study I propose to examine four questions: 1. What is the moral judgment on sterilization being made today by the pope, the bishops and the Church's theologians? 2. What is the proper way of making a moral judgment about sterilization and —by extension—other medical ethical questions? 3. What is the authority of the Church to make pronouncements in the field of morals? 4. Practically, what is the Catholic hospital in the U.S. to do about sterilization, given both the teaching of the pope, bishops and theologians and the practical situation I have described?

Notes

1. The account of the document's release is from *Origins*, 6, n. 3 (June 10, 1976), 35. The text was subsequently published in *L'Osservatore Romano*, December 11, 1976. Press comment at the time related the publication to compulsory sterilization in India. See *The New York Times*, December 12, 1976.
2. See *Hospital Progress*, 57, n. 3 (March 1976) for several articles on the implications of PL 93-641, the most recent federal legislation.
3. *The New York Times*, May 9, 1976. See also Leslie Aldridge Westoff, "Sterilization," *The New York Times Magazine*, September 29, 1974.

1.
Church Teaching on Sterilization

The practice of sterilization is not new.[1] The court eunuch who looked after the king's harem is a familiar figure in biblical and other ancient literature. In fact the most practicable form of permanent sterilization known to the ancient world was castration of the male. The anatomical information and surgical techniques that would have made possible the permanent sterilization of the female were not available.

The ancients did, of course, have crude forms of contraception, some of which were thought to have a temporary sterilizing effect, and there are references from time to time to "poisons of sterility" in Christian literature, apparently referring to these contraceptives, and all the references are condemnatory.[2]

The possibility of surgical sterilization for the control of fertility is not, however, a very old one. If one looks at the *Theologia moralis* of St. Alphonsus Liguori,[3] who died in 1787 but whose works continued to appear in numerous editions during the nineteenth century, one will find no discussion whatever of surgical sterilization as we know it. What one does find is a discussion of the morality of castrating singers for Church choirs —a practice not unknown in St. Alphonsus' time and even well into the nineteenth century. Curiously, St. Alphonsus does not reject the practice, although he reviews the opinions of moralists who think it wrong and calls their opinion "more probable." But the opinion of moralists who thought the practice permissible to improve the quality of Church music and provide a good living for the singers is described as "probable" and the point is made that the Church in fact tolerated the practice.

Church tradition was also aware of the early condemnation

of castration for religious reasons, such as it had been practiced by Origen, who made himself a eunuch for the Kingdom of God.

I mention these somewhat bizarre problems to make the point that the setting in which the sterilization question arose in moral theology was in terms of the liceity of mutilation. The decision was that it is not permissible to mutilate oneself, as Origen had, for religious reasons; but it was not so clear that mutilation was ruled out completely, if the motivation was partly religious, as in the case of the Church singers.

Of course moralists did recognize the permissibility of mutilating a part of the body for the good of the whole, e.g., by amputation, although there is a curious silence in St. Alphonsus about medicine and surgery in this context. But for the moment I merely note that the question of the *castrati* is discussed under the heading of mutilation and that the principle of bodily totality does not seem to be enough to explain or justify the castration of healthy male singers. There is no discussion of sterilization performed to protect the life of a woman which would be threatened by pregnancy.

The silence of moralists on therapeutic sterilization is not mysterious. The workings of the human reproductive system were not well understood until at least the second quarter of the nineteenth century, when von Baer published his discovery of the female ovum in 1827.[4] And despite the fact that Fallopius had described the tubes which bear his name in the sixteenth century, and van Leeuwenhoeck had discovered the male sperm in 1677, basic reproductive facts were simply unknown until the nineteenth century. Combine that with the fact that antiseptic surgery and anesthesia were not developed until the middle of the nineteenth century by Morton and Long for anesthesia and Lister for antisepsis, and it becomes clearer why modern surgical sterilization is not discussed by moralists. It was in 1834 that James Blundell suggested the sectioning of the fallopian tubes, but it was only between 1880 and 1910 that successful techniques of tubal ligation were developed.

That produced a different kind of moral evaluation.

The first attention to surgical sterilization seems to have

come from canonists who had to deal with the problem of sterility and impotence as possible impediments to matrimony. John Noonan has found a description of surgical sterilization in Cardinal Pietro Gasparri's canon law text on matrimony from 1894, but Gasparri limits his discussion to the problem of a possible marriage impediment. There is no discussion of sterilization among the major moralists of the nineteenth century. It is not until the first decades of the twentieth century that moralists began to write about surgical sterilization.

When they saw the procedure as contraceptive, their opinions were condemnatory, and in this they were but following an opinion of the Holy Office of May 22, 1895. The Holy Office was asked:

> Whether the practice is permissible either actively or passively of a procedure which intentionally proposes as an express purpose the sterilization of the woman?

The Congregation responded in the negative.[5]

Sabetti and Barrett, who cite this response, explain the condemnation not in terms of mutilation but in terms of contraceptive effect, which they find opposed to the primary purpose and good of matrimony, i.e., children, to the purpose of the matrimonial contract, to the purpose of the seed, and therefore contrary to the natural law, so that it can in no way be justified.

The position of Sabetti and Barrett is consistent with the traditional condemnation of contraception and also with the natural law doctrine which flourished under Leo XIII after the publication of the encyclical *Aeterni Patris* on the revival of Thomism in 1879. However, I think it is important both to note the shift from the older treatment of sterilizing surgery as mutilation to such surgery as contraception and to appreciate the historical situation in which the discussion began. Two factors are to be considered: one, the purpose for which surgical sterilization was used, and the other, the population question. We begin with a word about the eugenic use of sterilization.

In this connection, the development of techniques of vasectomy is instructive.[6] The early technique was developed at the Indiana State Reformatory by Dr. Harry C. Sharpe, using reformatory inmates as his experimental subjects. The purposes for which these techniques were employed were clearly eugenic. Sterilizations had also been carried out in Pennsylvania— without benefit of any legal authorization—apparently by a superintendent who wished to deliver his male inmates from self-abuse. Whatever the motivations of the first practitioners of eugenic sterilization, the movement gained ground rapidly after Indiana passed in 1907 a law providing for the involuntary sterilization of the mentally defective. The U.S. Supreme Court in *Buck vs. Bell* in 1927 declared such laws constitutional, with the ringing dictum of Mr. Justice Holmes that "three generations of imbeciles are enough." At one point twenty-seven states had laws providing for involuntary eugenic sterilization. Many such laws are still on the books.

The program of eugenic sterilization that was carried on in Germany under the Nazi regime beginning in 1933 is still remembered. The involuntary sterilization of thousands of men and women for eugenic reasons reached its peak in the 1930's, but the movement was underway earlier, perhaps as a result of the social Darwinism that had its origins in the nineteenth century.

The point is that the popes' moral evaluation of the new surgical techniques for the sterilization of both men and women had its origins in a climate which is regarded today even in legal circles as inimical to human freedom. The scientific arguments advanced for eugenic sterilization are recognized today as largely unfounded, despite the fact that the Supreme Court and many state legislatures presumably acted on that basis.[7]

There was another factor too: the population problem.

In his monumental study of the moral and canonical aspects of contraception, John Noonan has noted the relationship, often expressed, between declining population levels and opposition to contraception. Such arguments appear in the late nineteenth century in France, for example, after the debacle of the Franco-Prussian War.[8] Society—both Church and state —had a need for children which became another argument against contraception, one explicitly cited by bishops in Belgium, France and Germany in the period between the Franco-Prussian War and World War I—precisely the period when the eugenic sterilization movement was growing. In the period between 1880 and just prior to World War II, the birth rate declined in almost all Western European and North American countries to less than twenty per thousand, and England, Switzerland and Sweden just before World War II had net rates of reproduction of less than one, while Belgium and France in 1939 had rates slightly over one. Noonan comments:

> Western society seemed to be seeking stability of population and achieving it. In most countries this achievement appears to have been through contraception.[9]

Malthus' warnings had apparently been taken seriously over a period of many years.

But many countries perceived their population situation as a national threat. I have already mentioned France. The German Nazis and the Italian Fascists attempted to increase the populations of their respective countries, and I noted the eugenic dimension of their efforts.

Perhaps these indications are enough to suggest the climate in which the modern discussion of sterilization, especially through surgical techniques, arose. The Holy See condemned in eugenic sterilization what it properly viewed as the violation of the natural rights of those who were being involuntarily sterilized, even though the techniques were more sophisticated than castration. Sterilization by cutting or tying the fallopian tubes for contraceptive purposes was condemned as well, although it is important to note the circumstances, so different from our own in concern for population, in which the prohibition of contraception was restated. It should be noted too that Rome did not reject sterilization as punishment for crime. But it was in a generally disapproving climate that there occurred the earliest modern discussion of surgical sterilization to prevent even a pregnancy that would be life-threatening or at least seriously health-threatening to the mother.

The condemnation of eugenic sterilization took its most solemn form in the encyclical *Casti Connubii* of Pius XI in 1930. The same condemnation was repeated by Pius XI, Pius XII, and Paul VI, and by Roman Congregations.[10] These statements extend the condemnation to contraceptive and eugenic sterilization, but not always to punitive sterilization. They also make it clear that sterilization for therapeutic reasons can be permissible under the principle of double effect.

Sterilization was treated, except for contraceptive sterilization, as a form of mutilation, and moralists applied their usual rules. Or at least they tried. Mutilations are permissible for the good of the whole, under what Pius XII called the "principle of totality," the theological tradition said. Or sterilization might be the unavoidable side-effect of quite legitimate procedures such as prostate surgery or a hysterectomy demanded by some pathology of the reproductive system. These latter cases are called "indirect" sterilizations, because the primary intention is not sterilization but the treatment of the pathology of the reproductive system.

But neither the popes nor the moralists applied the principle of totality to the reproductive system itself. They did not recognize the legitimacy of sterilizing, if the pathology was located outside the reproductive system and the threat to life or health would arise only if a pregnancy occurred. It seemed easy enough to say that there is simply no such thing as an unavoidable pregnancy, except perhaps in the case of rape. In that case precautions against an unwanted pregnancy were permitted so long as they were not clearly abortifacient. The moralists, and the pronouncements of the Church authorities which they were following, explained this stance by declaring that the reproductive system, unlike other bodily organs, is ordered not to the good of the individual who possesses it, but to the good of the species. Thus the principle of totality may not be invoked but only the principle of double effect. Pius XII spoke to that effect in 1953.[11]

With the development of the anovulant pills in the 1950's, the same pope extended his prohibition of contraceptive sterilization to include temporary sterilization induced by the pill. Thus sterilization, whether produced by surgery or by drugs, whether permanent or temporary, whether of the male or the female, was proscribed when done for eugenic, contraceptive and even for therapeutic reasons, unless the sterilization was only the indirect effect of a procedure which had other direct therapeutic effects. Punitive sterilization, however, was still defended. That was the state of the discussion when Pius XII died in 1958.

Since the death of Pius XII and the election of Pope John XXIII, a great discussion has taken place in the Church on the meaning of marriage and the morality of regulating births. In the following pages I turn to several positions that have been taken on sterilization. I have tried to choose authors whose views are broadly representative of Church teaching, and I have also tried to present evidence drawn from a number of countries and language groups.

In March 1963, Pope John XXIII created a commission to study the question of birth control. The study commission was continued and enlarged by Pope Paul. I will turn below to its recommendations, but the task may be simpler if we treat Pope Paul's position first.

The pope's comment on the work of the commission, and the key to his own position, can be found in n. 6 of the encyclical *Humanae Vitae* (1968):

> The conclusions at which the commission arrived could not, nevertheless, be considered by us as definitive, nor dispense us from a personal examination of this serious question; and this also because, within the commission itself, no full concordance of judgments concerning the moral norms to be proposed had been reached, and above all because certain criteria of solutions had emerged which departed from the moral teaching on marriage proposed with constant firmness by the teaching authority of the Church.[12]

The encyclical then goes on to describe four characteristics of conjugal love, i.e., that it must be human, total, faithful and exclusive, and fecund. While the pope acknowledges the need for responsible parenthood, his conclusion is:

Nonetheless the Church, calling men back to the observance of the norms of the natural law, as interpreted by their constant doctrine, teaches that each and every marriage act must remain open to the transmission of life.[13]

The encyclical recognizes the legitimacy of using rhythm to regulate births, but of sterilization it says:

Equally to be excluded, as the teaching authority of the Church has frequently declared, is direct sterilization, whether perpetual or temporary, whether of the man or of the woman.[14]

Generally, since the teaching of *Humanae Vitae* is a restatement of the teaching of Pius XI and Pius XII, the encyclical does not provide lengthy arguments for its position. But there is one facet of the argument that is touched upon. In defending the use of rhythm while at the same time forbidding the use of artificial means of birth control, the pope writes:

In reality, there are essential differences between the two cases; in the former, the married couple make legitimate use of a natural disposition; in the latter they impede the development of natural processes. It is true that, in the one and other case, the married couple are concordant in the positive will of avoiding children for plausible reasons, seeking the certainty that offspring will not arrive; but it is also true that only in the former case are they able to renounce the use of marriage in the fecund periods when, for just motives, procreation is not desirable, while making use of it during the infecund periods to manifest their affection and to safeguard their mutual fidelity. By so doing they give proof of a truly and integrally honest love.[15]

The point to note in this paragraph is that it distinguishes between the moral and the immoral on the basis of a "natural process," i.e., on the basis of reproductive biology. And obvious importance is attached to the opportunity afforded by the use of rhythm to make abstinence an expression of conjugal love.

Briefly, I mention too another series of arguments, mostly on the basis of negative consequences, offered in *Humanae Vitae*. The pope fears that artificial birth control would open the road to conjugal infidelity and the general lowering of morality. Fear is expressed of a lowering of respect for women: men will become careless of the physical and psychological equilibrium of women and make of women instruments of selfish enjoyment rather than respected and beloved companions.

Moreover, Pope Paul fears the power that would be placed in the hands of public authorities if they seek to remedy population problems by immoral means and thus invade the most private sector of conjugal intimacy. On the basis of these grave consequences, the pope reaches the following conclusion:

Consequently, if the mission of generating life is not to be exposed to the arbitrary will of men, one must necessarily recognize insurmountable limits to the possibility of man's domination over his own body and its functions, limits which no man, whether a private individual or one invested with authority, may licitly surpass. And such limits cannot be determined otherwise than by the respect due the integrity of the human organism and its functions, according to the principles recalled earlier, and also according to the correct understanding of the "principle of totality" illustrated by our predecessor Pope Pius XII.[16]

The encyclical then has sought to define the limits of a person's licit intervention in the processes of one's own body, and it has sought those limits in the natural biological processes themselves, which the pope has described as grounding the natural moral law.

I need hardly say that the teaching of *Humanae Vitae* is

the authoritative view of the pope; it is shared too by bishops and theologians. I have not attempted to count heads or to determine the extent to which the encyclical's doctrine has been accepted. In the review of various views on sterilization being given here, it is enough to say that the teaching of the pope and the reasons offered in support of it are accepted by significant numbers of people in the Church. But there are other views, and I turn now to them.

In the turbulence which followed the publication of *Humanae Vitae* in 1968, the work of the papal commission to which the encyclical was reacting has not received much attention. The substance of its reports has, however, been published.[17] From the various published documents, I wish to comment only on what pertains to the question of sterilization.

The report adopted by the majority of the commission says this about sterilization:

> Sterilization, since it is a drastic and irreversible intervention in a matter of great importance, is generally to be excluded as a means of responsibly avoiding conceptions.[18]

While this is hardly a ringing endorsement, it must be noted that what is "generally to be excluded" might, given the proper circumstances, be permitted. The position of the commission therefore represented a modification of the position taken by the Holy Office in 1936 and 1940, which declared direct sterilization intrinsically immoral.[19]

How did the commission arrive at its position? The teaching of the Holy Office, which was repeated by *Humanae Vitae*, was that sterilization is intrinsically evil *ex defectu juris*, i.e., because it was an action which the agent had no right to perform. In 1953 Pius XII had explained at some length why the principle of totality ought not to be invoked when the danger to the total human life and health arose not from some pathology of the reproductive system but from the threat posed by a future pregnancy. The pope held that since pregnancy is voluntary, the principle of totality could not apply.[20]

In brief, the argument of the commission runs this way:

The fundamental principle is that of responsible parenthood. In the discharge of their responsibility the couple may find the regulation of conception necessary. To this end some intervention in physiological processes, ordained to the essential values of marriage and first of all to the good of children, is to be judged according to the fundamental and objective principles of morality.

A right ordering toward the good of the child within the conjugal and familial community pertains to the essence of human sexuality. Therefore the morality of sexual acts between married people takes its meaning first of all and specifically from the ordering of their actions in a fruitful married life, that is, one which is practiced with responsible, generous and prudent parenthood. It does not then depend upon the direct fecundity of each and every particular act. Moreover, the morality of every marital act depends upon the requirements of mutual love in all its aspects. In a word, the morality of sexual actions is thus to be judged by the true exigencies of the nature of human sexuality, whose meaning is maintained and promoted by conjugal chastity, as we have said.[21]

The reader will note, I think, that a fundamental difference of approach exists about human dominion over biological processes and whether and to what extent those processes can be considered *morally* normative. The reader will also note that the commission insists that there are objective criteria for the moral evaluation of interventions in physiological processes. The commission wrote:

The objective criteria are the various values and needs duly and harmoniously evaluated. These objective criteria are to be applied by the couples, acting from a rightly formed conscience and according to their concrete situation.[22]

There are also objective criteria as to the means to be employed. Thus Vatican II altogether rejected abortion or procedures that are thought to be abortifacient. Then there follows the comment that sterilization is generally to be excluded because it is a drastic and irreversible intervention. As to other means the commission writes:

> Moreover, the natural law and reason illuminated by Christian faith dictate that a couple proceed in choosing means not arbitrarily but according to objective criteria. These objective criteria for the right choice of methods are the conditions for keeping and fostering the essential values of marriage as a community of fruitful love. If these criteria are observed, then a right ordering of the human act according to its object, end and circumstances is maintained.[23]

First, then, the action must correspond to the nature of the person and his acts so that the meaning of procreation is kept in the context of true love.[24] Second, the means chosen must have an effectiveness proportionate to the necessity of averting a new conception temporarily or permanently. Third, since every method, even abstinence, has certain negative effects, the means chosen must carry the least possible negative effects for the concrete couple. Fourth, the means chosen must be considered in the light of what is available to the couple in their specific situation, including its economic factors.[25]

Thus, the commission insists, couples properly instructed are to make their decision "not arbitrarily, but as the law of nature and of God commands; let couples form a judgment which is objectively founded, with all the criteria considered."[26]

The commission also devoted a section to indicating what it considered the continuity of its position with the previous teaching of the Church more profoundly understood. Noting that the rhythm method has been approved by the popes, despite the fact that the use of it separates the reproductive from the other aspects of marital acts, the commission wrote:

> The tradition has always rejected seeking this separation with a contraceptive intention for motives spoiled by

egoism and hedonism, and such seeking can never be admitted. The true opposition is not to be sought between some material conformity to the physiological processes of nature and artificial intervention. For it is natural to man to use his skill in order to put under human control what is given by physical nature. The opposition is really to be sought between one way of acting which is contraceptive and opposed to a prudent and generous fruitfulness, and another way which is in an ordered relationship to responsible fruitfulness and which has a concern for education and all the essential, human and Christian values. In such a conception the substance of tradition stands in continuity and is respected.[27]

I conclude this review of the commission's stand with another citation, this one from a document on "pastoral approaches" prepared for the pope by some of the bishop members of the commission:

What has been condemned in the past and remains so today is the unjustified refusal of life, arbitrary human intervention for the sake of moments of egoistic pleasure; in short, the rejection of procreation as a specific task of marriage. In the past, the Church could not speak other than she did, because the problem of birth control did not confront human consciousness in the same way. Today, having clearly recognized the legitimacy and even the duty of regulating births, she recognizes too that human intervention in the process of the marriage act for reasons drawn from the finality of marriage itself should not always be excluded, provided that the criteria of morality are always safeguarded.

If an arbitrarily contraceptive mentality is to be condemned, as has always been the Church's view, an intervention to regulate conception in a spirit of true, reasonable, and generous charity does not deserve to be, because if it were, other goods of marriage might be endangered. So what is always to be condemned is not the regulation of conception, but an egoistic married life, refusing a creative opening-out of the family circle, and so refusing a truly human—and therefore truly Christian—married love. This is the anti-conception that is against the Christian ideal of marriage.[28]

Although the commission's view did not win the pope's acceptance, I have dealt with it at length both for the approach to the natural law which it employs, which is rather different from that of the encyclical, and also for its view of the relationship between its viewpoint and that of the tradition. In the words of a theologians' report to the study commission, "Man is the administrator of life and consequently of his own fecundity."[29] The commission, therefore, sees human physiology as being at the disposal of human reason and not as a norm-giver to it, even in matters of reproduction. The commission also has a rather different view of human sexuality than has often been found in the Christian tradition, and it stresses the interpersonal dimensions of sexual love, even as it insists on the ordering of love to a prudent and generous fecundity. And, finally, the commission claims to preserve the *values* traditionally proclaimed by the Church's teaching authority, even though it recognizes that it proposes new *norms* with respect to contraception.

With these contrasting views in mind, I turn to some current theological writing on the subject of sterilization. I have tried to locate materials which would reflect not only the work of American theologians and practice in this country, but also that of other places.

In the November 1974 issue of the German periodical *Stimmen der Zeit*,[30] Franz Böckle, professor of moral theology in the University of Bonn, published an article on "Ethical Aspects of Voluntary Sterilizing Operations."

Böckle's treatment is in two parts. The first treats sterilization as a mutilation, and the second deals with sterilization as contraceptive. As to the first, Böckle notes that the principle of totality has traditionally been applied. When a physical pathology is involved the case is obvious enough and is really not in dispute. But Böckle points out that the principle has been extended to justify the voluntary castration of men guilty of sexual misconduct. The totality then must therefore include more than just the physical totality of the body and extend at least to psychic totality as well.[31]

Böckle also refers to the use of the principle of totality when prophylactic sterilization was under consideration. He mentions in particular the situation of the nuns in the Congo, in which the use of sterilizing pills was justified by theologians held in high esteem in Rome on the ground that contraception was prohibited *only* when sexual relations were voluntary, and in the Congo situation they were most involuntary. Hence the principle of totality could be invoked to avoid the consequences of involuntary sexual relations. This reading of the 1958 allocution of Pius XII on the principle of totality is thoroughly ingenious and representative of a legal model of morality in the hands of real experts.

Böckle has another situation too. He distinguishes between "infertility" and "sterility." "Infertility" means that a woman is unable to carry a child to viability. "Sterility" means that a conception is not possible. Böckle then argues that the moral order is violated only by the destruction of a healthy fertility. Therefore in cases of infertility a directly sterilizing operation does not violate the moral order but instead is therapeutic. Böckle notes that after consultation among German moral theologians, this opinion was included in a book of principles and counsels in marriage matters for German physicians and he calls it a *sententia probata*, which I take to mean not only probable but officially approved. And he concludes:

On the basis of this fact we could say that the official teaching of the Catholic Church does not oppose a medically indicated sterilizing operation in concrete cases.[32]

But Böckle has more. He then suggests that the principle of totality can be extended even to the marriage, so that a husband could be sterilized in place of the wife. Böckle says that in the relationship of the individual to society the individual human being can never simply be sacrificed to human society. But, he argues, the fertility of a marriage is in a certain degree an indivisible whole related to the unity and indissolubility of the marriage itself. Therefore, when there are weighty reasons for not sterilizing the woman, and where the age and life situation of the man would make it a responsible action, the principle of totality could be applied to the marriage and the husband vicariously sterilized for his wife. All this, of course, assumes that fertility as defined has been destroyed. Böckle is of the opinion that even this latter case is not contrary to the position of *Humanae Vitae* on contraception.

Then Böckle turns to sterilization as a form of contraception. Noting the widespread disagreement among German Catholics with the position of *Humanae Vitae* (sixty-one percent disagreed in a poll) and the action of various bishops' conferences in pointing to the possibility and the obligation of the faithful to make their own decision in conscience—an event without parallel in modern Church history—Böckle proceeds to a critique of the encyclical's position. In brief, Böckle rejects the notion of "intrinsically evil acts" that underlies the encyclical's position on contraception and which in turn is grounded in the encyclical's position on the normative character of biological processes as willed by God. Böckle's formulation of a moral rule is this: "It is immoral actively to exclude birth from sexual love *(Hingabe)*, unless avoiding conception is indicated by weighty reasons and abstinence would be injurious to the well-being of the couple."[33]

Given sufficient grounds for contraception, the choice of means depends on the health and the personal values of the couple.

Böckle then applies this analysis to sterilization:

Whoever holds with *Humanae Vitae* that every artificial contraceptive act is intrinsically evil must reject also every sterilization for simply prophylactic reasons. But whoever, counter to *Humanae Vitae*, treats contraception as not an evil in every case (and this could be a considerable part of the bishops and theologians) must treat sterilization as a "last resort" for an indicated prevention of contraception. The moral judgment will conscientiously weigh the positive and negative consequences for the integral good of the person. Where a lasting avoiding of children is indicated, there the sterilization could be included in the same consideration.[34]

Böckle, like the papal commission, holds that the choice of contraceptive methods, including sterilization as a last resort, must be made by the couple according to objective criteria. And he ends his article with the statement:

Where contraception by drugs is tolerated by Catholic hospitals, it follows that sterilizing operations as a last resort in a necessary and lasting prevention of conception should be permitted as well.[35]

Employing rather different moral criteria and methods, Böckle has arrived at a quite different conclusion from the encyclical's. It is difficult to know how widely his ideas are shared in Germany, especially with regard to prophylactic sterilizations. He does refer in the course of his discussion to recent synods, including the recent German synod, in which a position similar to his on birth regulation seems to be at work.[36]

The lines of quite different positions are appearing by this time, so I will summarize more briefly other discussions, largely for the purpose of indicating the spread of the point of view they represent.

Even prior to the publication of *Humanae Vitae,* Eugéne Tesson had published an examination of a number of situations in which sterilization, either permanent or temporary, might be considered, as well as some situations in which the anovulant pill might be used for other than directly sterilizing purposes, e.g., the control of irregular cycles, etc.[37]

Tesson describes the situation in which Catholic moralists concluded that it was legitimate to perform a hysterectomy to remove a uterus that *would* pose a problem if a pregnancy occurred but which is not otherwise a health problem. The case of the uterus after multiple Caesarean sections is an example. Although not all theologians agreed, the opinion of Gerald Kelly, S.J., who defended a hysterectomy in such a case, was widely accepted.

Tesson presses the case further. If a hysterectomy could be performed in such cases, could not a physician achieve the same effect by tying the woman's tubes, a much less drastic procedure? Tesson agrees that a tubal ligation and sterilization in such a case is justified, either by surgery or the use of the anovulant pill. What has come to be called an "isolation procedure" of this sort is justified by the argument that *qui maius potest, minus potest*, the sterilization being the less drastic action.

In Canada the practice of Catholic hospitals can be measured by the codes of ethics that some of them have adopted. In London, Ontario, St. Joseph's Hospital adopted a "Policy Manual for a Committee To Advise on Requests for Obstetrical/Gynaecological Sterilization Procedures."[38] The policy is this:

A. There are medical instances in which a tubal ligation may be considered as a final procedure to be used in the total treatment of a woman who is judged unable to support a future pregnancy.

B. The only reason for allowing sterilization in this hospital is the presence of a pathological condition in the woman.

C. Only those medical indications will be considered which pose a permanent major threat to the life and health of a woman.

The moral underpinning of this position is explicitly the principle of totality, understood as the physical totality of the woman, which would be threatened by a future pregnancy. The policy modifies the position of *Humanae Vitae* and Pius XII by extending the principle of totality to the reproductive system, but it does not envision sterilization for purely contraceptive reasons.

The Ottawa General Hospital[39] performs sterilizations for obstetrical, gynecological, surgical, and psychiatric reasons without prior committee review, provided that the indications are verified in a consultation with colleagues in the field. Ottawa does seem to have periodic post-operative review. It is of some interest that among the indications is one for the case of a mother with a retarded, psychotic or epileptic child, when the woman must still act as mother and wife. The policy statement says: "In certain cases a sociological evaluation is almost indispensable to carry out a decision." Thus the principle of totality has been extended.

Two hospitals in Toronto[40] have adopted policy statements based on two basic values: (1) the commitment of the hospitals to their Roman Catholic status and to the obligations which result from this status vis-à-vis their constituency; (2) the respect of the hospital for the individual religious and moral convictions and family relationships which influence the patient's decision concerning the number of their children and the time in their marriage when they decide to opt for permanent forms of family planning. The policy is a statement about the conditions under which the hospital will *cooperate*. That framework is noteworthy.

In cases of conflict between these two sets of values, the hospitals will decide whether or not to cooperate on the basis of: (1) informed consent of the patient; (2) marital status, age of the couple and the number of children; (3) assurance that the medical, psychological or socio-economic indications warrant limitation in the size of the family on a permanent basis; (4) a signed statement by the couple that it is their conviction that they are making a conscientious decision.

The policy requires that persons to be sterilized in these hospitals be thirty years of age, and with at least three children, if the decisive arguments are socio-economic. Single persons will not be sterilized unless there is a strict medical counter-indication to pregnancy.

It is hardly necessary to point out the increasingly broad grounds, especially socio-economic ones, which are indicated here. But there is also explicit reference to a rather new factor: the individual religious and moral convictions of the person or couple requesting sterilization. The influence of discussions about moral and religious liberty since Vatican II is obvious. It should also be noted that Ontario has a health-care plan which involves the hospitals.

The precise moral ground for these policies is not indicated, but there is reason to think that in addition to the principle of totality, which may be operative in some cases, there are at least two other considerations. One is a conflict of parental obligations. On this point the bishops of Canada expressed themselves in their statement on *Humanae Vitae*[41] when they noted a possible "clear conflict of duties, e.g., the reconciling of conjugal love and responsible parenthood with the education of children already born or with the health of the mother." It is possible, although I am unable to document it, that the judgment in some cases may simply be that permanent means of contraception are needed in view of some other and broader principle of morality than the principle of totality.

With that I turn to the position taken by Father Charles E. Curran in his article "Sterilization: Roman Catholic Theory and Practice"[42] and by Richard McCormick, S.J. Father Curran discusses the position of the popes on sterilization and various interpretations put upon it by theologians, including the famous Congo situation. He also mentions again punitive sterilization, and yet another situation of the incompetent female who cannot provide for her hygienic needs or who is in danger of being impregnated. Sterilization for hygienic reasons he regards as indirect sterilization since its purpose is not contraceptive at all but hygienic, and thus it falls well within traditional limits, provided that important questions of adequate and informed consent are met. Sterilization in the case of the incompetent in danger of being impregnated Curran regards as parallel to the Congo situation and also falling well within traditional limits, again if important questions of informed consent are satisfied.[43]

Generally, however, Curran wished to handle the whole subject in a rather different framework. For one thing Father Curran would extend the principle of totality to include the good of the whole person, not just his physical being. The good of the whole person would include his relationship to his family, community and the larger society. Curran also knows of the opinion that totality might be extended to the marriage.

But in addition to the principle of totality, Father Curran would invoke the principle of man's stewardship over his sexuality and his generative organs. Rather than consider sterilization in terms of mutilation, with its traditional emphasis on totality, and indirect and direct effects, Curran would consider it in the same basic terms as contraception. Thus surgical sterilization and the use of anovulant pills belong in the same discussion, since both are sterilizing and the difference is only in duration of effects. Whenever contraception can be justified on a permanent basis, Father Curran would see the moral possibility of a sterilization, provided that the usually permanent and irreversible effects are understood. The weight of the reasons needed to justify a sterilization under the principle of stewardship should be in proportion to the permanent effects of the procedure. Richard McCormick, S.J., has published what is fundamentally a similar opinion.

The Code of Ethical and Religious Directives for Catholic Health Facilities of course repeats the statements of *Humanae Vitae* prohibiting any direct sterilization. The Code was adopted in 1971 by an overwhelming majority of the American bishops (232 to 7) and has been promulgated in a number of dioceses.

In a curious development, however, Father Anthony Kosnick, who is a member of the Advisory Committee to the Bishops' Committee on Health Affairs of the U.S. Catholic Conference, did a survey of dioceses in the U.S. The responding dioceses represent those in which a large portion of Catholic health facilities are found. In his report[44] on procedures being followed with regard to Directive 20 on sterilization, Father Kosnick writes:

The matter is urgent for medical men who insist that concern for the welfare of the total person as well as the practice of responsible medicine requires recourse to sterilization procedures in some instances. Diverse interpretation of this Directive 20 has led to widely divergent practices and applications with regard to sterilization procedures in Catholic hospitals. In one diocese it was indicated that prior to the promulgation of the Directives a policy had been in effect that permitted sterilizations for medical purposes, including psychiatric reasons, under the principle of totality.[45]

Confusion of course followed the apparently restrictive policy declaration of Directive 20. But what is telling in Kosnick's report is his description of sterilization committees set up in Catholic hospitals and at work without complications or difficulties for a year in early 1973! Note that these are explicitly sterilization committees, which must mean that, despite Directive 20, tubal ligations for medically indicated reasons are being and have been done since the new Code was published in a significant number of American dioceses. Just how many Kosnick does not say, but he has enough information to provide three different models for such committees. I omit the details. What is significant is that a policy approved 232 to 7 by the American bishops' conference has not been strictly observed in American Catholic hospitals. The indications for sterilizations, however, seem to be limited to medical ones. Policy in the U.S. is apparently stricter than in Canada.

In summary then, the development of surgical techniques of sterilization and the Church's reaction to them has taken place since the 1890's. While castration of Church singers had been defended and practiced for centuries, the problem had been considered one of mutilation by moralists. But when sterilization became available as a contraceptive technique, it was forbidden along with other forms of contraception. Both *Humanae Vitae* and the recent Roman reply are restatements of this doctrine, which is explained as an application of the natural law.

But other opinions have gained adherents in the Church. The papal commission and many contemporary theologians urge that contraception and sterilization can be morally justified under some circumstances.

That raises two additional questions: (1) How does one go

about making a moral judgment about sterilization—or anything else? (2) What is the authority of Church officials to make pronouncements about moral questions?

The next two chapters deal with these questions in turn.

Notes

1. See Jonas Robitscher (ed.), *Eugenic Sterilization* (Springfield: Charles C. Thomas, 1973): J. Robitscher, "Introduction: Eugenic Sterilization: A Biomedical Intervention," pp. 3-16; J. Paul, "State Eugenic Sterilization History: A Brief Overview," pp. 25-40.
2. See John T. Noonan, Jr., *Contraception: A History of Its Treatment by the Catholic Theologians and Canonists* (Cambridge: Harvard, 1965).
3. *Theologia moralis*, ed. by Michael Heilig (Malines: P. J. Hanicq, 1852), esp. vol. 3, p. 99.
4. See Arturo Castiglioni, *A History of Medicine*, trans. and ed. by E. B. Krumbhaar (New York: Knopf, 1941); and Theodore Cianfrani, *A Short History of Obstetrics and Gynecology* (Springfield: Thomas, 1960); B. E. Finch and Hugh Green, *Contraception Through the Ages* (Springfield: Thomas, 1963); Larry L. Langley (ed.), *Contraception* (Benchmark Papers in Human Physiology) (Stroudsburg, Pa.: Dowden, Hutchinson and Ross, 1973).
5. Cited in A. Sabetti, S.J. and T. Barrett, S.J., *Compendium theologia moralis*, 22nd ed. (New York: Pustet, 1915), p. 250. See Noonan, *Contraception*, p. 429; and T. J. O'Donnell, S.J., "Sterilization," in *New Catholic Encyclopedia*, XIII, pp. 704-5.
6. See note 4.
7. See *Relf v. Weinberger* 372 US 1196ff. (1974) and *Wyatt v. Aderholt* 368 Fed Supp 1382 (1974); and also Robitscher. HEW regulations on the use of federal funds for sterilization were published in the *Federal Register*, 39 (1974), 4730-33 and 13872-73.
8. Noonan, p. 414.
9. *Ibid.*, p. 410.
10. The materials are assembled by John C. Ford, S.J., and Gerald Kelly, S.J., *Contemporary Moral Theology*, II, pp. 315-37, 2 vols. (Westminster: Newman, 1963). See also *Litterae encyclicae de matrimonio christiano*, ed. by F. Hürth, S.J., Textus et Documenta, series theologica, n. 25 (Rome: Gregorian University Press, 1953) for text and commentary on *Arcanum* (Leo XIII, 1880) and *Casti Connubii* (Pius XI, 1930). See also *The Human Body*, ed. by the Monks of Solemnes (Jamaica Plains: Daughters of St. Paul, 1960) for various papal statements.

11. Text in Ford and Kelly, p. 322-24. See also 1958 address cited at pp. 341-42. *The Human Body*, p. 279, n. 501.
12. *Humanae Vitae*, USCC edition, n. 6.
13. *Ibid.*, n. 11, with footnote to *Casti Connubii*, p. 560, cited in Hürth, pp. 48-49, and to Pius XII, *Allocution to Midwives*, October 29, 1951, AAS 43 (1951), p. 853, cited in Hürth, pp. 90-91. The 1951 allocution is also in *The Human Body*, n. 268, p. 160.
14. *Humanae Vitae*, n. 14, with note to *Casti Connubii*, p. 565, and to the Decree of the Holy Office, Feb. 22, 1940 (DB 2283), and to *Roman Catechism*, II, 8.
15. *Humanae Vitae*, n. 16.
16. *Humanae Vitae*, n. 16, with note to AAS, 45 (1953), pp. 674-75 (Allocution to Urologists), and AAS, 48 (1956), pp. 461-62 (Allocution to Congress on Sterility and Fertility).
17. *The Birth Control Debate*, ed. by Robert G. Hoyt (Kansas City: National Catholic Reporter, 1968).
18. *Ibid.*, p. 93.
19. Texts in Hürth, pp. 114-16.
20. Allocution to Urologists, Oct. 8, 1953; *The Human Body*, nn. 500-501.
21. Hoyt, p. 87-88.
22. *Ibid.*, p. 92, with note to GS, nn. 50 and 87.
23. *Ibid.*, pp. 93-94.
24. Note to GS, n. 51.
25. Hoyt, p. 94.
26. *Ibid.*
27. *Ibid.*, pp. 90-91.
28. *Ibid.*, pp. 106-107.
29. *Ibid.*, p. 74.
30. Franz Böckle, "Ethische Aspekte der freiwilligen operativen Sterilisation," *Stimmen der Zeit*, 99 (1974), 755-60.
31. The principle of totality has been analyzed by John M. Cox, *A Critical Analysis of the Roman-Catholic Medico-Moral Principle of Totality and Its Applicability to Sterilizing Mutilations*, a dissertation from the Claremont Graduate School (Ann Arbor: University Microfilms, 1972). Cox concludes that contemporary circumstances require a modification of the ban on direct sterilizations.
32. Böckle, p. 756.
33. *Ibid.*, p. 759.
34. *Ibid.*
35. *Ibid.*, p. 760.
36. *Ibid.*, p. 759.
37. E. Tesson, "Discussion morale," *Cahiers Laennec*, 24 (1964), 64-73.

38. St. Joseph's Hospital, London, Ontario, 1973.
39. "Indication for a Sterilization, Committee of Hospital Morality, Ottawa General Hospital" (n.d.).
40. "Suggested Medico-Moral Guidelines," St. Joseph's Hospital, Toronto, Sept. 27, 1974. The same are in force at St. Michael's Hospital.
41. Text in Hoyt, pp. 165-74, n. 26 at p. 172.
42. *Linacre Quarterly*, 40 (1973), 97-108. See Richard McCormick, S.J., "Vasectomy and Sterilization," a reply to a letter of L. L. deVeber, M.D., *Linacre Quarterly*, 38 (1971), 7 and 9-10.
43. Curran, pp. 100-101.
44. Anthony R. Kosnick, "The Present Status of the Ethical and Religious Directives for Catholic Health Facilities," *Linacre Quarterly*, 40 (1973), 81-90.
45. *Ibid.*, p. 85. Directive 20 reads: "Procedures that induce sterility, whether permanent or temporary, are permitted when: a. they are immediately directed to the cure, diminution, or prevention of a serious pathological condition and not directly contraceptive (that is, contraception is not the purpose); and b. a simpler treatment is not reasonably available. Hence, for example, oophorectomy or irradiation of the ovaries may be allowed in treating carcinoma of the breast and metastasis therefrom; and orchidectomy is permitted in treatment of carcinoma of the prostate." Directive 18 reads: "Sterilization, whether permanent or temporary, for men or for women, may not be used as a means of contraception."

2.
Right and Wrong and
Natural Law

I

A thesis that I want to defend throughout this study is that medical-ethical questions are first of all *ethical* questions, and not simply matters having to do with the social behavior and graces of physicians.[1] Within a religious context they are questions of moral theology or Christian ethics. That is to say that such questions are not merely questions for moral philosophy, but instead pertain to man's relationship with God.

Of course ethics has to do with making normative judgments about the rightness or wrongness of a prospective course of action. Since I will be dealing with natural law, I will discuss the question of norms and normative judgments. But before I do that, I think there is a need to look very briefly at some aspects of the ethical task that may shed light on the questions before us.

Consider, for example, that theological ethics is concerned not simply with discovering the appropriate rules which govern a particular moral problem, but with the whole situation of man before God. It is the Christian conviction, stated with great force in Paul's letter to the Romans, that every human person stands before God as a sinner. There was a dispute between Catholics and Protestants over the depth and extent of the damage done by human sinfulness. Here it will be enough to note that Catholics today take more seriously than was sometimes the case their own theological dictum that humanity has been "wounded" by sin in such a way that human intelligence has been darkened and human freedom weakened. Bernard Lonergan, for example, has recently translated the catechism's darkened intellect and weakened will into a "scotosis" of the intellect and an "antecedent moral impotence,"[2] but the meaning is unchanged.

To acknowledge that human beings are sinners living in a sinful world is to lay the groundwork for some appropriate modesty in making claims for one's ethical insights. The redemptive work of Jesus Christ has no doubt overcome sin and sinfulness, but the full realization of Christ's victory over sin will not come within human history. The moralist must not forget that. Sin is a component of the present human situation.

When Catholics have spoken of "sin," they traditionally have thought of the violation of a rule. Morality is, in fact, often defined as conformity to a rule.[3] I would describe such a model of morality and sin as a legal one.

Many Catholic theologians today are aware that a legal model of sin is not enough.[4] Sin is something more than simply the violation of a law or rule. Sin has to do with relationships between persons, with relationships between human persons and God. That means that a great deal of the language used for generations by Catholics to describe and classify sins is inadequate. Consider for example the way in which Catholics were taught to distinguish "mortal" sin and "venial" sins.[5] Perhaps the easiest example had to do with matters of justice. If one stole a small amount, the sin was only venial, but if one stole a great deal, the sin was mortal. The point on the scale at which a venial sin passed over into a mortal one was placed variously by various theologians and depended on the time and place of the misdeed. Most moralists held that all sexual sins were serious ones.

The difference between a mortal sin and a venial sin was, however, enormous. Moralists taught that one who committed mortal sin had cut off his relationship with God, turned his back on an eternal destiny with God and was doomed to an eternity of separation from God in wretchedness. Venial sin, on the other hand, while an offense against God and a weakening of one's relationship with him, did not destroy a relationship with God and did not entail such terrible and eternal consequences. Mortal sin and venial sin were clearly different *kinds* of things.

Moral theology had the task of carefully classifying the various rules one was obliged to follow in order to distinguish those which implied mortal sin if they were violated from those which did not. Such classifications were especially important for priests who heard confessions and had to make a judgment on whether serious sins had been committed.

A legal model of sin has many advantages. It tends to produce clear-cut judgments not only about what is right and what is wrong but even about the degree of the rightness or wrongness.

But the model also produced some incongruous results. It produced, at least at times, a cycle of sin, confession, and forgiveness, followed by sin, confession, forgiveness, etc. Any priest of experience who dealt with the recidivist anxious to confess sins and be absolved from habitual wrong-doing must have suspected that something was the matter with a view of things that had reduced the biblical drama of sin and conversion to a frantic cycle of habitual sin and equally habitual absolution.

The legal model also produced a great multiplicity of sins, since the violation of many laws and rules could accompany any human undertaking. Thus the priest who omitted even one of the little hours of the Divine Office was told that he had sinned gravely,[6] as was the priest who omitted the prescribed cleansing of the chalice at Mass.[7] Thus the offending priests found themselves consigned to perdition along with murderers and bandits.

I think it is not too much to say that theologians who were prepared to put violations of the Mass rubrics and cold-blooded murder in the same ethical category had not sufficiently considered the implications of their judgment. It is really impossible to imagine that separation from God and wretchedness for eternity were the fate of every priest who omitted even once a part or even all of the Divine Office, even if his reasons were thoroughly unworthy.

Problems of this sort have led Catholic theologians to reexamine the notion of sin, and especially the notions of "mortal" and "venial" sins. What has emerged is a different way of thinking about sin, which stresses less the violation of rules and more the violation of personal relationships that underlie the rules. Thus, for example, one finds writing about mortal sin as a "fundamental option," just as faith and conversion are a kind of fundamental option that gives direction and orientation to a life as a whole. Just as conversion produces a "new" person, with a "new" view of himself and the world, so sin which is truly "mortal" produces a fundamentally altered person with quite a different view of and relationship to himself and the world. The model is not a legal one; the role of rules is clearly secondary to the relationships between persons that the rules describe. And it becomes clearer how what the tradition has called venial sins are not incompatible in the same person with a fundamental option for God, just as in human relationship love is not incompatible with misunderstandings and disagreements—even rather serious ones.

Admittedly this "relational" model is not as tidy as the legal one. It is not so simple a matter to describe and classify all the possible actions that might reflect the fundamental option against God which is mortal sin. The task of the confessor in making judgments about the spiritual state of his penitents is more complex and more likely to focus on the longer term relation than on single acts.

All this may seem somewhat remote from the natural law and its relationship to medical ethics. But I would like to suggest that the attitude one takes toward moral rules will depend in significant measure on one's notion of what sin is and how it affects one's judgments. And it will depend on one's notions about the uses of moral rules in determining what a sin is and whether a particular sin is serious or not. Hopefully this brief discussion can remind us that there is more to ethics than discovering and attempting to apply the rules.

I have been dealing with sin and its effects and the way in which sins were described and classified in traditional moral theology. Let me add just a word now about the other side of the story: the effects of conversions and growth in moral virtue.

Bernard Lonergan[8] insists that religious conversion alters one's world view, transvalues one's values and makes a change in one's antecedent willingness to do the good one apprehends.

The religiously converted person "sees" the world in a different way, according to Lonergan. His perception of the moral good will be different from that of someone who is not converted. If religious conversion has been really thoroughgoing, it implies a moral conversion as well, i.e., a shift in values away from mere satisfaction for one's self to what is really worthwhile. And one will not only *see* the good, but will in fact *do* the good.

Lonergan suggests that if one wants to know what is truly good, one should consult the conscience of the truly virtuous person, because it is such a person who will recognize the genuinely good from its counterfeits.

One could find similar views on the implications of religious conversion in Karl Rahner. Both of these prominent voices in contemporary Catholic theology regard themselves as disciples and interpreters of Thomas Aquinas. Like Aquinas, they regard Christian ethics or moral theology not simply as a matter of describing and classifying sins, but as concerned with the human person converted to God and growing in the Christian life, in the love of God and the neighbor through God's grace.

The mention of grace leads me to a final preliminary remark. It is the observation that the grace of God is not increased in value by creating an artificial scarcity. Unlike commodities of various sorts, the grace of God is beyond price precisely because it is *God's* grace. It is a part of Catholic belief that God gives his grace to every human being during his lifetime in order that every person might be saved. God's grace is not limited to members of the Church, or to Americans, or to members of the white race, or to people of whom we approve.

The fact that God's grace is offered and may well be accepted by people who are not members of the Christian Church community, let alone of the Catholic Church, is another bit of groundwork for some appropriate modesty when believers undertake serious reflection on ethical problems. If Lonergan and Rahner are right on the effects of religious conversion, they also imply that religious and moral conversions are not necessarily limited to Church members, or to Christians, or to Catholics.

With these reflections on sin and sinfulness, the results of religious and moral conversion, growth in moral virtue and the presence of God's grace, I turn now to the more specific question of natural law.

II

The first part of most textbooks in moral theology is devoted to "fundamental moral theology," and among the questions raised there is that of the sources of moral theology. The texts typically respond that the sources are two: reason and revelation. The natural moral law is the product of reason. If one inquired where revelation was to be found, the answer was that it was found in scripture and tradition.

The First Vatican Council explained the need for revelation this way:

> It is to be ascribed to this divine revelation that such truths among things divine as of themselves are not beyond human reason can, even in the present condition of mankind, be known by everyone with facility, with firm assurance, and with no admixture of error.[9]

Catholic moralists have sometimes attempted to identify moral obligations that could not have been known without revelation.[10] But clearly most moral matters that are said to be revealed fall in the category of things revealed in order that they may be known with facility, with firm assurance, and with no admixture of error and not because they are in principle inaccessible to human reason. Moreover, it is clear enough that many moral problems confronted by Christians today are not even mentioned in the scriptures.

In a recent study of "Scripture and the Christian Ethic" Raymond Collins reached five conclusions: first, ethical teaching is an integral part of the gospel message for each of the New Testament authors; second, New Testament authors borrowed liberally from a variety of sources, so that there is an openness and a pluralism in New Testament ethics: there is no single ethical view in the New Testament; third, formal norms predominate over concrete norms, even though there are plenty of concrete ethical directives that are meant to concretize the formal norms; fourth, agapeic love is the single thread that links together the ethical teaching of the various New Testament authors, but even this is presented by them in various ways; and fifth, the New Testament authors present their various ethical views in a theological context. Father Collins writes:

> Ethics are Christian in so far as the living of the ethical life is a way of being a disciple of Jesus. Love is a Christian virtue in so far as it is a matter of loving as Jesus loved. Ethics are Christian in so far as to love as Jesus loved is to respond to the command of the Father and to love with the love of the Father himself. The ethical life is a necessary response to the presence of the kingdom of God among us. This quality underscores the urgency of the ethical demand as it relates to the Christian . . . Finally there is a pneumatic dimension to Christian ethics in so far as the Spirit of God, given to the children of God, is the power wherewith they are enabled to respond to the ethical demand. The Spirit is himself both the gift of power and the source of demand. The command of the Lord Jesus, the presence of the kingdom and the gift of the Spirit are so many ways of saying that there is a Christian motivation for living the ethical life.[11]

Natural law has played a vital role in Christian ethics as Christians sought to supply the concrete moral norms that were needed in facing specific situations.[12] The role of natural law has been a continuous one in the Catholic tradition, from the time of Ambrose and Augustine to the developments of the middle ages that culminated in the work of Thomas Aquinas, through the elaborations of the Spanish jurists of the sixteenth and seventeenth centuries to the renaissance of natural law in the neo-scholasticism of the nineteenth and twentieth centuries. Much of the teaching of the Catholic Church on social, political, and economic matters in the last century or more has explicitly appealed to the natural law for its authority. And the teachings of recent popes on medical-ethical questions have similarly appealed to the natural law as their warrant. The very first footnote of the encyclical *Humanae Vitae* appealed to the natural law teaching of popes since Pius IX in 1846. John XXIII elaborated a whole program for world peace in his encyclical *Pacem in Terris* on the basis of the natural law and Vatican II followed the lead of the popes.

Christians did not, of course, invent the idea of the natural law.[13] They found it already in use among the Stoics, and the Roman jurists found natural law useful in their dealings with a great diversity of peoples and cultures being brought together under a single system of Roman law. One of those lawyers, Ulpian, defined the natural law as "that which nature has taught all animals." One thinks at once of such basic and "natural" functions as reproduction and nutrition that man has in common with lower forms of animal life.

But there is another definition of natural law that also comes from antiquity. Cicero defined natural law as "what human judgment has not engendered, but an innate power has implanted." The differences between these definitions are important. Both are found in medieval Catholic theology. If Ulpian's definition is accepted, then what nature has taught all animals is morally normative. A moral obligation arises from the very physical structure of the "natural" act. If Cicero's definition is accepted, then what is obligatory arises not from the physical structure of the act, but rather from the prescription of some innate power. To make a long story short, St. Thomas held that that innate power is reason. And with that recognition comes the question whether natural law is something proper to human beings alone or something humans share with other animal forms.

The tension between these two approaches to natural law can be found in Aquinas himself, and I cannot hope to review here the volumes that have been written trying to settle just what St. Thomas thought. A careful review of St. Thomas' thinking that appeared in 1974 concluded that Thomas was ambiguous and used Ulpian's definition for reasons that are not clear.[14] But what does not seem to be ambiguous is that for St. Thomas human reason is what distinguishes man from other animal forms, and it is human reason that participates in the divine reason. The natural moral law, which is the product of human reason, shares in the eternal law, which is the product of God's wisdom.

Perhaps all this reads like little more than a historical curiosity. But in the field of medical ethics, it is not.

For one thing, the natural law doctrine of St. Thomas affirms that the natural moral law is the product of human reason. But St. Thomas insists that the natural law is not something human beings are born knowing. It is the product of experience on which reason deliberates.[15]

What Aquinas called the primary precepts of the natural law are very general indeed: do good and avoid evil, for instance. More particular moral precepts are only secondary at best. That too is important, because Aquinas insists that while the primary precepts of the natural law are known by everyone and are everywhere the same, other moral obligations based on natural law do not have the same qualities and some of them can change.[16]

These statements are important. There is no "code" of natural law available to be consulted. The natural law is man's reason reflecting upon experience and arriving at an understanding of moral obligation. There is no suggestion in Aquinas that any special group has privileged reasoning that gives them, but not others, access to the natural law. Secondly, except for its primary precepts, which are extremely general, the natural law for Thomas Aquinas is neither so well known nor so absolutely immutable as some recent discussions of the natural law might lead us to suppose. Even human nature can change, according to Aquinas,[17] so there is room for growth and at least some change in St. Thomas' own view of the natural law.

For medical ethics there is another and very important point. Aquinas does write of man's natural inclinations as that upon which reason deliberates in arriving at the natural moral law. The sense in which St. Thomas uses the notion of "inclinations"[18] is hotly disputed, but what is certain is that what gives moral force to the natural law is not the physical arrangement of things—in reproduction for example—but the dictate of the moral reason as it deliberates upon the human experience in reproduction. Law for Aquinas is always an ordinance of reason. Reason grounds moral obligation. Among contemporary Catholic theologians, there exists a diversity of views about the meaning and usefulness of natural law. Karl Rahner, for example, holds that the natural law can be discovered only by a transcendental reflection upon human knowing and willing and that "nature" is a kind of limit, which will be recognized only when humans try to go beyond it. But Rahner holds that within the limit of "nature," thus understood, humans are free to and even obliged to manipulate their own being. Rahner has also proposed a theory of moral instinct that can reveal the values at stake in complex moral analysis, in particular in those areas in which the manipulation of the human heritage, e.g., by genetic engineering, is involved.[19]

Even in the recent encyclicals of the popes the notion of natural law has been rapidly transformed from the classic natural law found in a universal and God-given order, which underlies the program of *Pacem in Terris*, to the more personalist conception of natural law found in Paul VI's encyclical on the development of peoples.[20]

But in spite of the range of views on the natural law, Catholic theologians continue to insist that a relationship between man's nature, especially his reason, and his behavior can and does determine a moral norm. Reason can determine what ought to be done.[21]

III

This point can be further illustrated with reference to sterilization. Various documents of the Roman magisterium and the teaching of the theologians who explained and supported it held that sterilization is an intrinsic moral evil. Writing in 1936,[22] the Holy Office declared that sterilization is intrinsically evil *ex defectu juris in agente*, i.e., because the agent has no right to perform such an act.

This language and the tradition of moral analysis of which it is a part claim Thomas Aquinas as their author. To say that an act is intrinsically evil is to say that the very act itself is morally evil, that the moral evil does not arise from an immoral intention on the part of the agent or from some combination of circumstances that have rendered an otherwise licit act depraved. It is to say also, of course, that no worthy intention and no set of circumstances will transform an act that is intrinsically evil into one that is morally upright. A moral agent may, of course, be mistaken in his/her judgments about an action, and thus more or less inculpable, but nevertheless, the tradition asserted, intrinsically evil acts were always objectively wrong.[23]

Moral theologians held some acts to be evil of their very nature and others similarly intrinsically good: blasphemy was often cited as intrinsically evil and the love of God as intrinsically good. But other actions were said to be evil by defect of right in the agent. Here both the examples and the problems are more numerous: adultery, murder, and theft are examples of actions of this sort. The defect of right is what qualifies adultery, for example, as a moral evil, while loving sexual intercourse between husband and wife is a morally good act. Similarly, the taking of the goods of another is theft unless the taker is invested with the right either by purchase, or by the provisions of law, or, in extreme need, by an overriding right to the goods in order to survive. Aquinas holds that in the latter case all goods are held in common, i.e., the right to survive takes precedence over the right to private property. The same argument held that not all killing is murder, but that *unjustified* killing is murder and thus evil *ex defectu juris*. But killing might be justified in cases of self-defense or the defense of another or in the case of capital punishment by public authority for the common good.[24]

A third category of evil acts were those the commission of which carried with them an unjustifiable danger of committing sin. Examples would be reading books that would endanger one's faith, or performing immodest acts which would lead to acts of unchastity.

A number of Catholic writers in the last decade or more have pointed to the abstractness of this kind of analysis.[25] They argue that it seems to assume that certain kinds of acts can be adjudged evil apart from their actually being performed by a moral agent. And there is the further point that traditional doctrine, even in Aquinas, did see certain situations in which acts evil *ex defectu juris* might in fact be obligatory. Granted that Aquinas was faced with problems from biblical examples of God's ordering such actions (e.g., the slaying of Isaac by Abraham), the point is that he did not hesitate to see that even "intrinsically evil" acts could in fact be done at times.[26]

Still other Catholic writers have studied the principle of double effect.[27] Although their studies have taken various forms, the conclusion is that to speak of *moral* evil, as the tradition does, is to speak of a situation in which "physical" or "ontic" or "pre-moral" evil has been caused *without proportionate justification*. There is a sense in which every human action falls into the category of acts with double or even multiple effects. The classic principle of double effect demanded (among other things) a proportion between the good to be accomplished and the evil that was permitted but not intended. Here an example might be taken from war, which was said to be justified in certain cases, *provided* that the good to be accomplished, e.g., the vindication of justice or the preservation of liberty, was not outweighed by the destruction and killing that war brings. In the judgment of many, the war in Vietnam failed the test of proportion and was therefore unjustifiable.

If the example of war clarifies at least the notion of the proportion that the moral tradition demanded between the good to be sought and the evil to be permitted, then the contemporary discussion extends the principle to *any* action. Here again a traditional category is helpful. The tradition spoke of physical evil, which it distinguished from moral evil. Contemporary writers often prefer to speak of "ontic" or "pre-moral" evil. Their point is that every human action carries with it some element of such evil, even if it is simply the "evil" inherent in choosing one course of action and thus excluding another; or the "evil" in exercising my liberty and thus making a certain space/time unavailable to another person.[28] Each action that I perform is therefore clouded to some degree by the fact that it brings evil inevitably into the world.

If I continue to act despite this sobering realization, it is because I judge that on balance the good I seek to accomplish by my actions outweighs the evil that is also produced by them. The heart of moral decision-making, then, is the judgment I must make about the proportion between the pre-moral evil my actions will bring into the world and the good that my actions are to achieve. If there is in fact no good proportionate to the pre-moral or ontic evil, then my action is *morally* evil; but my action does not pass into the properly moral realm until this judgment has been made. Until an agent is involved and acting, it is not possible to use moral categories at all; one can at best speak of actions only in the abstract.

Authors who write in this vein take pains to point out that the judgment about the proportion between pre-moral or ontic evil and the good that I seek to achieve is not merely a subjective one. Traditional Catholic doctrine has stressed the function of reason in making moral decisions precisely of this kind: one thinks at once of the principle of double effect and its application in the case of the just war doctrine. Moral judgments about the war in Vietnam, for example, are not merely subjective.

It is also made clearer, in the judgment of these writers, that in deciding to act I have taken moral responsibility for all the foreseeable effects of my actions. It is not necessary to speak of the ontic evil my actions bring into existence as somehow "outside of" or "beyond" my intention. From a moral point of view I am fully responsible for the injury or death I inflict upon an assailant in defending myself. What morally differentiates physical injury or even killing in such an instance from battery or murder is the judgment that a proportion does exist between the good I seek to achieve in defending myself and the ontic or pre-moral evil which is the injury or death of the assailant. Injuring or even killing the assailant is thereby morally justified without ceasing to be recognized as an evil, and I acknowledge that in defending myself by the use of violence, I have foreseen and thus intended injury and even death to the assailant. The proportion between pre-moral or ontic evil and the good to be achieved appears if we consider the moral difference between the surgeon who uses a knife to remove diseased tissue and thus promote the life of his patient, and the criminal, whose use of the knife is immoral precisely because there is no proportionate reason to justify the ontic evil (fear, injury, death) he produces.

Arguing along these lines, Peter Knauer can then conclude that to speak of "intrinsic evil" is simply to speak of "moral evil"; that is, it is to speak of the case in which there is no proportion between the good to be achieved and the concomitant ontic evil.[29] To speak of the "moral" while considering an action in the abstract, before the agent has made a judgment about the multiple effects of his action, is to be premature. What distinguishes moral evil from ontic evil is the inescapable responsibility of the agent to minimize evil and thus to insure that there in fact exists a proportion between the ontic evil his action will produce and the good he seeks. It is proper to speak of "intrinsic" evil in the case of murder, theft or unjustified sexual intercourse, because the moral quality of the act is not dependent merely upon the good intentions of the agent: the proportion between good and evil in the concrete case can be assessed and judged objectively.

With these things in mind, it is possible to review what the tradition discussed in chapter one has said about sterilization. The judgment has been that sterilization is intrinsically evil *ex defectu juris in agente*. In the scheme of object, intention and circumstances proposed by St. Thomas, sterilization is ruled immoral in the very object of the act, apart from the intention of the agent or the circumstances. The moral object (sterilization) is said to be wrong not from the very nature of the act, like blasphemy, or from the danger of sin, like the commission of immodest acts, but from a defect of right on the part of the agent. The same sort of judgment has been made against adultery, murder and theft.

The argument that supports this judgment appeals to the purpose of the reproductive system for evidence. The reproductive faculties do not exist for the good of the individual human person but for the good of the species. Therefore, to subordinate the reproductive system and its use to the good of the individual is to injure the human race as a whole, something that no one has the right to do. The argument could be pressed further to urge the danger of the extinction of the race that could follow from the subordination of the good of the species to the good of the individual or couple; and it could be developed and given a more directly religious aspect by noting that the designs of the Creator are found in the arrangements of nature, so that to do violence to the natural purposes of things is to do violence to what God has willed. The judgment that sterilization is "intrinsically evil" from a defect of right in the agent summarizes a whole array of arguments pointing to the evils that would result to the human species, and thus implicitly at least to every human being and to God, if sterilization were judged permissible.

It is undeniable, I think, that sterilization does bring evil into the world. But the weakness of the line of argument that I have summarized is its abstractness. The flat generalization that sterilization is always, everywhere and under all circumstances forbidden by the moral law short-circuits the process of making a moral judgment, because it does not permit the agent to ask whether there are or might be reasons which would justify bringing about that evil, reasons of such weight that a proportion does or could exist between the evil that the act will produce and the good that the agent seeks to achieve.

Unquestionably evils do result from sterilization. If the sterilization is surgical and permanent, it involves a violent intrusion into the body of either male or female, with the risks to life and health that any surgical intervention involves. The cutting of the *vas deferens* in the male or the fallopian tubes of the female is not only violence to the body, but it suppresses the functioning of the reproductive system as a whole: the sterilized male or female can no longer procreate. The loss of reproductive function too is an evil, both for the individual and (arguably at least) for the human race. But all of these are what the tradition has called "physical evils" and what more recent discussions have called "pre-moral" or "ontic" evils.

What seems dubious in the traditional analysis is its supposition that there can exist no proportionate reasons to justify the performance of sterilization. By casting the argument into a conflict between the good of the individual and the good of the species, the tradition has sought to preclude any good of the individual that might be offered. But such an argument cannot stand as a moral judgment, since the nub of moral argument is precisely the weighing of the proportion between the admitted pre-moral or ontic evils that sterilization involves and the goods that the moral agent pursues in performing a sterilization. The good of the species is not decisive *tout court* and neither is reproductive biology.

Therefore it does seem to make a difference whether the sterilization is performed to prevent a pregnancy that would seriously jeopardize the life and health of a woman (both important goods surely) or whether the sterilization was performed under government auspices to reduce the number of prospective welfare clients.[30] I would argue that a sterilization procedure that is to preserve the life and health of the mother which otherwise would be threatened by a pregnancy offers a clear example of goods to be sought (life, health, the preservation of a marriage relationship, care of children already born, etc.) that can and do in many cases outweigh the evils which sterilization entails, and therefore can be morally permissible. The same procedure performed under government auspices on minor women without adequate information and their consent is quite another matter, in which the evils arising from the violation of the personal and civil rights of the welfare recipients combine with the evils inherent in the sterilization procedure itself to compel the judgment that the action was immoral, because there was no proportionate reason to justify allowing such a combination of evils. Sterilization for contraceptive purposes would similarly require solid justification.

This line of argument is in the natural law tradition that stresses the function of reason in weighing the proportion between the good to be sought and the evils that will accompany it. It is consistent with the treatment of other moral issues like killing, sexual intercourse, and the taking of another's property, because it distinguishes between cases in which a proportionate reason exists and others in which it does not. Just as not all killing is judged murder, not all sexual intercourse adulterous, and not every taking a theft, so not every suppression of human fertility can be judged immoral.

It may be objected that the strength of the traditional position in Catholic thought is its very intransigence. Since it permits no exceptions whatever, it gives steadfast witness to the good of human fertility and to the principle that human beings are only the stewards with limited dominion over the body God has given them. To suggest that there may be some situations in which sterilization can be morally justified is to open the door to sterilization on demand, to the spread of a contraceptive mentality, and ultimately to the scourge of abortion.

I reply that intransigence cannot be a substitute for moral responsibility. If it is correct to say that the morality of an action is to be judged by whether or not a proportion exists between the ontic evil it produces and the counterbalancing good being sought, then it is not enough simply to proclaim that being moral means adherence to a moral principle, whatever the evils that may result. To do so is to substitute adherence to the principle for one's own responsibility. To be sure, the evils of moral irresponsibility, loss of esteem for the value of human life, and widespread abortion are things that must be weighed in the balance when a judgment is to be made. The demands of a sound public policy are a weighty concern. But it is not possible to assert *a priori* that any one of these prospective evils excludes a judgment that proportionate reasons could exist for performing some sterilizations. But the argument does emphasize the fact that the more serious and numerous the evils which may result from an act, the greater the good required to be truly proportionate.

I have been arguing that natural law is the product of human reason reflecting upon experience. It is not innate in us; it does not exist in codified form. The primary precepts of the natural law seem very close to the fundamental moral intuition that good is to be done and evil is not to be done. What is good and what is evil must therefore be determined by deliberation upon experience. What is decisive in those deliberations is the judgment whether a proportion exists between the ontic or premoral evil that accompanies any human action and the good the agent seeks by acting. While moral generalizations are useful in making such judgments, they cannot be a substitute for them.

Therefore the process of formulating specific natural law obligations is not something done once and for all, but is instead the continuous task of responsible human deliberation. I have argued that such deliberation would indicate that sterilization can at times be morally approved.

For Christian ethics, natural law is therefore an indispensable source of moral wisdom. But it is also the work of the same human beings whose knowledge and freedom have been infected by sin. We have no assurance that even conversion and the profession of the Christian faith will totally eradicate from each of us or from the community the effects of sin. Granted then both the need and the usefulness of the natural law, the moral deliberation that produces it is still that of sinful men and women or at best of men and women still growing in a life of virtue.[31] Growth in understanding of moral matters is entirely compatible with a notion of natural law, and in fact seems to be demanded by it.

Yet the human person deliberating on moral obligations does not exist in lonely isolation. He or she is a member of a community, perhaps of several communities. Before our reflections are done we must ask what the religious community has to say to the believer as he or she seeks to know what is right and what is wrong.

Notes

1. See Joseph Fletcher, *Morals and Medicine* (Boston: Beacon Press, 1954), p. xix; Paul Ramsey, "The Nature of Medical Ethics," in *The Teaching of Medical Ethics*, ed. by Robert M. Veatch, Willard Gaylin, and Councilman Morgan (Hastings-on-Hudson: Institute for Society, Ethics and the Life Sciences, 1973), pp. 14-28; Daniel Callahan, "Bioethics as a Discipline," *The Hastings Center Studies*, 1:1 (1973), 66-73; Robert M. Veatch, "Medical Ethics: Professional or Universal?" *Harvard Theological Review*, 65 (1972), 531-59; Arthur J. Dyck, "Ethics and Medicine," *Linacre Quarterly*, 40 (1973), 182-200.
2. *Insight: A Study of Human Understanding* (Student edition; New York: Philosophical Library, 1958), pp. 191-92 and 627-30.

3. See, for example, Marcellino Zalba, S.J., *Theologiae moralis summa, I: Theologia moralis fundamentalis* (Madrid: Biblioteca de Autores Cristianos, 1952), p. 151.

4. For what follows, see, for example, Louis Monden, S.J., *Sin, Liberty, and Law* (New York: Sheed & Ward, 1965).

5. On mortal and venial sin, see Bruno Schüller, "Zur Analogie sittlicher Grundbegriffe," *Theologie und Philosophie*, 41 (1966), 3-19.

6. John A. McHugh, O.P., and Charles J. Callan, O.P., *Moral Theology: A Complete Course*, 2 vols. (New York: Wagner, 1930), II, p. 587.

7. McHugh and Callan, *Moral Theology*, II, p. 671.

8. I have dealt with the views of Lonergan and Karl Rahner in "Faith and Christian Ethics in Rahner and Lonergan," *Thought*, 50 (1975), 247-65. On conversion, see Lonergan's *Method in Theology* (London: Darton, Longman & Todd, 1972), pp. 237-43.

9. First Vatican Council: Dogmatic Constitution on the Catholic Faith (1870), chap. 2, in *The Teaching of the Catholic Church*, ed., by J. Neuner and H. Roos; revised by Karl Rahner (Staten Island: Alba House, 1967), n. 32.

10. See, for example, Joseph Fuchs, S.J., *Theologia moralis generalis* (2 vols. 2nd ed.; Rome: Gregorian University Press, 1963), I, p. 89. Fuchs mentions the obligation of loving God in a supernatural manner, living in Christ and in grace, the obligation of believing, etc.

11. Raymond Collins, "Scripture and the Christian Ethic," in the *Proceedings of the Catholic Theological Society of America*, 29 (1974), pp. 215-41; citation at pp. 240-41.

12. See Vernon Bourke, *St. Thomas and the Greek Moralists* (Aquinas Lecture, 1947) (Milwaukee: Marquette University Press, 1947); Michael Wittman, *Die Ethik des hl. Thomas von Aquin: in Ihrem systematischen Aufbau dargestellt und in ihren geschichtlichen, besonders in den antiken Quellen erforscht* (Munich: Hueber, 1933); Heinrich Rommen, *The Natural Law*, trans. by Thomas R. Hanley, O.S.B. (St. Louis: B. Herder, 1947), esp. pp. 34-69.

13. See Odon Lottin, O.S.B., *Le droit naturel chez saint Thomas d'Aquin et ses predecesseurs*, 2nd ed. (Bruges: Beyaert, 1931); Jean-Marie Aubert, *Le Droit Romain dans l'Oeuvre de saint Thomas* (Paris: Vrin, 1955), in addition to the material in n. 12.

14. See Michael Bertram Crowe, "St. Thomas and Ulpian's Natural Law," in *St. Thomas Aquinas 1274-1974: Commemorative Studies*, ed. by Armand A. Maurer, C.S.B. 2 vols. (Toronto: Pontifical Institute of Mediaeval Studies, 1974), I, pp. 261-82. Crowe's conclusion that Thomas' use of Ulpian is "in the last resort, slightly puzzling" might be compared with Aubert's in *Le droit romain*, p. 99, or Lottin's in *Le droit naturel*, pp. 64-66. Aubert has argued in "Le droit naturel, ses avatars historique et son avenir" in

La vie spirituelle: Supplement, 81 (1967), 282-322, esp. pp. 298-302, that Thomas uses the notion of tendencies to make of natural law not something merely ideal, but something morally obligating in the real order. All the students of St. Thomas emphasize the medieval problem of reconciling apparently conflicting *auctoritates*, which Thomas did in the case of natural law by assigning Ulpian's "natural law" to what was common to both men and other animals, and to the "ius gentium" what was the specifically human product of reason. The problem of Thomas' use of tendencies is, therefore, in significant measure one of assigning the proper label. It does not seem to me to be necessary to tax Thomas with responsibility for an excessive physicism in formulating moral obligation, as does Charles E. Curran, *Contemporary Problems in Moral Theology* (Notre Dame: Fides, 1970), pp. 16-111.

15. Joseph T. C. Arntz, O.P., in "Natural Law and Its History," *Concilium*, n. 5 (1965), 39-57, and "Die Entwicklung des naturrechtlichen Denkens innerhalb des Thomismus," in *Das Naturrecht im Disput,* ed. by Franz Böckle (Düsseldorf: Patmos, 1966), pp. 87-120, has argued that for St. Thomas the natural law is only that which is *naturaliter cognitum*, i.e., known without ratiocination by a process of intellectual intuition. Lottin, *Le droit naturel*, pp. 72-73, had affirmed the contrary.

16. *Summa theologica*, I, II, 95, 5, *in corp.*

17. See the texts cited by Joseph Fuchs, *The Natural Law: A Theological Investigation*, trans. by H. Rickter and J. A. Dowling (New York: Sheed & Ward, 1965), p. 93.

18. See note 15.

19. See his "Naturrecht: Heutige Aufgaben," in *Lexikon für Theologie und Kirche*, VII, cols. 827-28. Rahner does know, however, of an *a posteriori* natural law as well. See *Theological Investigations*, I (Baltimore: Helicon, 1961), p. 299n. and "The Problem of Genetic Manipulation," in *Theological Investigations*, IX, pp. 225-521 on faith instinct.

20. The shift from the emphasis of *Pacem in Terris* (1963) on the order in nature which man is to discover and follow to that of *Populorum Progressio* (1967), in which the development of man himself has become the moral norm, is quite remarkable.

21. See Bruno Schüller, "La théologie morale peut-elle se passer du droit naturel?" in *Nouvelle Revue Théologique*, 88 (1966), 449-75, and "Zur theologischen Diskussion über die lex naturalis" in *Theologie und Philosophie*, 41 (1966), 481-503.

22. See text in *Litterae encyclicae de matrimonio christiano*, Textus et Documenta, series theologica, n. 25, ed. by F. Hürth (Rome: Gregorian University Press, 1953), pp. 114-15.

23. See M. Zalba, *Theologia moralis*, pp. 170-201; *Summa theologica*, I, II, 18.

24. See *Summa*, II, II, 64, 2 and 7; 66, 2.
25. See, for example, Joseph Fuchs, S.J., *Theologia moralis generalis*, 2 vols. (Rome: Gregorian University Press, 1968-69), I, p. 601; Louis Janssens, "Ontic Evil and Moral Evil," *Louvain Studies*, 4 (1972), 115-56. The issues dealt with here have been reviewed by Richard A. McCormick, S.J., in his "Notes on Moral Theology" in *Theological Studies*, 36 (1975), 85-100, and 37 (1976), 71-87, in the course of an extensive review of the literature.
26. See J. G. Milhaven, "Moral Absolutes and Thomas Aquinas," in *Absolutes in Moral Theology?*, ed. by Charles E. Curran (Washington: Corpus Books, 1968), pp. 154-85.
27. Joseph T. Mangan, S.J., "An Historical Analysis of the Principle of Double Effect," *Theological Studies*, 10 (1949), 41-61; J. Ghoos, "L'acte à double effet: Etude de théologie positive," *Ephemerides theologicae Louvaniensis*, 27 (1951), 30-52; Peter Knauer, S.J., "La détermination du bien et du mal moral par le principe du double effet," *Nouvelle révue théologique*, 87 (1965), 356-76; Cornelius van der Poel, "The Principle of Double Effect," in *Absolutes in Moral Theology?*, pp. 186-210; Peter Knauer, S.J., "The Hermeneutic Function of the Principle of Double Effect," *Natural Law Forum*, 12 (1967), 132-62.

An extended treatment of this crucially important discussion is beyond the scope of this study.
28. See a further discussion in Karl Rahner, "The Theology of Power," *Theological Investigations*, IV, trans. by Kevin Smyth (Baltimore: Helicon, 1966), pp. 391-409, esp. pp. 396-97.
29. P. Knauer, "The Hermeneutic Function," p. 138.
30. Such were the circumstances in cases brought to the federal courts in which welfare recipients or wards of the state were involuntarily sterilized. The issue of free and informed consent is, of course, related and morally important, and it suggests that an important public policy issue is involved here too. See *Relf vs. Weinberger*, 372 U.S. 1196 and *Wyatt vs. Aderholt*, 368 Fed Supp 1382.
31. Bernard Lonergan has captured this sense of the need for continuing growth in his notion of multiple and continuing conversions, including moral conversion. See note 8.

3.
Morals and the Magisterium

It would be impossible to turn the pages of the New Testament without being impressed by the importance of behavior in the Christian life. Behavior, or praxis or ethics—whatever name one chooses—is an integral part of being a Christian.[1]

It should come as no surprise then to learn that the Church, which has been given the task of preaching the gospel, should also find itself involved in giving directions and making decisions on moral matters. The gospel writers and Paul and James often addressed themselves to a variety of moral concerns. The Fathers and other Church authorities have done and are doing much the same thing to this day.

In the last couple of centuries there has been a great development of the theology of the teaching authority of the Church or *magisterium*, as it is often called. In the various divisions of the Church's task that theology has developed, the three-fold division of prophet, priest, and king, first applied to Christ, has come to be applied also to the work of the Church and thus we have another triad: *sacerdotium* (priesthood), *imperium* (ruling or royal office) and *magisterium* (teaching office or perhaps prophetic office, if we keep the parallelism with the offices of Christ). A great deal of the development of theology about the *magisterium* has taken place in the nineteenth and twentieth centuries.[2]

In its definition of papal infallibility, the First Vatican Council said that the pope "is possessed of that infallibility with which the Divine Redeemer willed that his Church should be endowed for defining doctrine regarding faith or morals. . . ."[3]

This teaching authority is exercised in what is called an "extraordinary" way in councils or other rare and especially solemn ways, or it can be exercised in "ordinary" ways, in the day-to-day teaching of those who hold the teaching authority. When they teach as revealed a matter of faith or morals and are in accord with one another and with the Roman pontiff their teaching is regarded as infallible.

Vatican II repeated verbatim what Vatican I had said about the papal teaching authority and it added the qualification that infallibility extended as far as the deposit of revelation extended, which is to be religiously guarded and faithfully expounded.[4]

The Council added that when the pope or the bishops teach in this way, "In matters of faith and morals, the bishops speak in the name of Christ and the faithful are to accept their teaching and adhere to it with a religious assent of soul."[5]

Vatican II's explanation of the term "deposit of faith" can be found in the Council's Constitution on Divine Revelation, which says:

> Sacred tradition and sacred Scripture form one sacred deposit of the word of God, which is committed to the Church. . . . The task of authentically interpreting the word of God, whether written or handed on, has been entrusted exclusively to the living teaching office of the Church, whose authority is exercised in the name of Jesus Christ. This teaching office is not above the word of God, but serves it, teaching only what has been handed on, listening to it devoutly, guarding it scrupulously, and explaining it faithfully by divine commission and with the help of the Holy Spirit; it draws from this one deposit of faith everything which it presents for belief as divinely revealed.[6]

The teaching of the Council on matters that are taught by the Church as divinely revealed seems clear enough. The Church draws her teaching from the deposit of faith by which textbook theology meant scripture and tradition, and it is the task of the teaching authority of the Church to explain and guard this deposit, not to make additions to it or modifications in it. This work of the teaching authority of the Church is aided by the Holy Spirit. What such teaching means is clear enough in matters of *faith*.

But the problem we are considering is of a different sort. I indicated that a large body of moral teaching has been elaborated by modern popes on a variety of social questions and also in the field of medical ethics. Warrant for such teachings has not been claimed by an appeal to divine revelation, but by an appeal to the natural law. An obvious question arises: What is the source of the authority claimed by the Church to teach matters that are acknowledged not to be contained in the deposit of revelation? And what are the limits and conditions of such teaching, which theology has described as "authentic but not infallible"? To say that it is authentic is to say that it is authoritative and demands assent. To say that it is not infallible means that either in principle or in fact such teaching is not the subject of an infallible pronouncement by the Church's teaching authority.

There are, I think, at least two ways of putting questions such as these. One way is to affirm with the Council that the charism of infallibility extends as far as the deposit of divine revelation extends, with the clear implication that it extends no farther; and then to ask by what authority the Church teaches matters not revealed and which it therefore cannot teach infallibly. Putting the question in that fashion implies that the deposit of revelation is something like a bank deposit: at least it contains a sum of things revealed which the Church can teach infallibly. Moral teachings of the Church which are not in that sum of things revealed are the problem. The usual way of putting this would be to assume that moral teachings like "Thou shalt do no murder" are much like doctrinal teachings such as "Jesus Christ is truly God and truly man." When the term "deposit of faith"[7] is used to imply that revelation is a sum of truths or propositions, then this way of putting the question seems natural enough.

But one might ask the question in a different way.[8] If what God has revealed in Jesus Christ is first and foremost himself, then the term "deposit of faith" surely refers to what God has revealed in Jesus Christ; but then revelation does not seem to be, primarily at least, a series of propositions. To be sure the Church has and does formulate statements of revelation, but it is not obvious anyway that the "deposit of faith" is a quantity of such statements on which the Church can draw as the need arises.

What the Church proclaims in her preaching and teaching is God's revelation of himself in Jesus Christ. This preaching has always been described as "putting on a new man" or as a "rebirth" and a "new way of life." It goes without saying that conversion and faith imply not only accepting truths but also a new mode of behavior.

From this perspective the question of the authentic noninfallible *magisterium* looks a bit different. Instead of teaching truths—moral truths—that are not contained in a deposit of revelation understood as a collection of propositions, the work of the authentic noninfallible *magisterium* would be to suggest the implications in practice of this new way of life which is an integral part of Christian faith.

In whichever way one puts the question, there does indeed remain a problem about the sources and the extent of the Church's teaching authority in morals, particularly when no claim is made that the moral teaching is revealed and when the admission is made that the moral teaching is derived from the natural law.

I now propose to review several understandings of the *magisterium* and morals.

I

The teaching of the Second Vatican Council reflects a body of doctrine about the *magisterium* that has been developed in the nineteenth and twentieth centuries. One of the clearest and most authoritative statements of that teaching can be found in two allocutions of Pope Pius XII, given in 1954. The pope undertook to review the duties of bishops in these two talks, and in doing so he divided their responsibilities in the familiar pattern of teaching, sanctifying and ruling, or following the offices of Christ as prophet, priest and shepherd-king.[9]

The pope's teaching can be summarized briefly: The Lord

entrusted the truth which he brought from heaven to the Apostles and to their successors the bishops.

> The Apostles are, therefore, by divine right the true doctors and teachers in the Church. Besides the lawful successors of the Apostles, namely the Roman Pontiff for the universal Church and the Bishops for the faithful entrusted to their care (cf. can. 1326), there are no other teachers divinely constituted in the Church of Christ.

> Others who teach in the Church do so by delegation from the pope or the bishops and as their associates. The bishops are to supervise the doctrine taught by those whom they have delegated by such measures as prior censorship of books and by monitoring lectures, books, classroom notes and the like intended for the use of students.

> In matters involving the salvation of souls, there is no teaching authority in the Church not subject to this authority and vigilance.[10]

In his second talk, Pope Pius turned to the priestly and pastoral offices of the bishops. I pass over the statements about the priestly office as not pertinent and turn to the pope's statements about the pastoral office.

It is in the context of the pastoral office, and—interestingly —not in the context of the teaching office, that Pius XII took up the question of the Church and the natural law. The pope said:

> The power of the Church is not bound by the limits of "matters strictly religious," as they say, but the whole matter of the natural law, its foundation, its interpretation, its application, so far as their moral aspects extend, are within the Church's power. For the keeping of the Natural Law, by God's appointment, has reference to the road by which man has to approach his supernatural end. But, on this road, the Church is man's guide and guardian in what con-

cerns his supreme end. The Apostles observed this in times past, and afterwards, from the earliest centuries, the Church has kept to this manner of acting, and keeps to it today, not indeed like some private guide or adviser, but by virtue of the Lord's command and authority. Therefore, when it is a question of instructions and propositions which the properly constituted shepherds (i.e., the Roman Pontiff for the whole Church and the Bishops for the faithful entrusted to them) publish on matters within the natural law, the faithful must not invoke that saying (which is wont to be employed with respect to the opinions of individuals): "the strength of the authority is no more than the strength of the arguments." Hence, even though to someone, certain declarations of the Church may not seem proved by the arguments put forward, his obligation to obey still remains. This was the mind, and these are the words of St. Pius X in his Encyclical Letter *Singulari Quadam* of September 24, 1912 (AAS 4 [1912] p. 658): "Whatever a Christian may do, even in affairs of this world, he may not ignore the supernatural, nay, he must direct all to the highest good as to his last end, in accordance with the dictates of Christian wisdom; but all his actions, in so far as they are morally good or evil, that is, agree with, or are in opposition to, divine and natural law, are subject to the judgment and authority of the Church." And he immediately transfers this principle to the social sphere: "The social question and the controversies underlying that question . . . are not merely of an economic nature, and consequently such as can be settled while the Church's authority is ignored, since, on the contrary, it is most certain that it (the social question) is primarily a moral and religious one, and on that account must be settled chiefly in accordance with the moral law and judgment based on religion" (*Ibid.* pp. 658, 659).[11]

This lengthy citation expresses with great clarity the position of Pius XII, which he expressly connects with the teaching of Pius X. Problems that pertain to the moral order "cannot be declared outside the authority and care of the Church."[12]

But note again that these problems are treated as falling within the *pastoral* and not the *teaching* authority of the Church and are expressly related by Pius XII to the jurisdiction of the bishop and to matters of Church discipline.[13]

The authority of the Church is grounded in the fact that the questions being addressed are "moral questions" and thus fall within the scope of the authority of the Church in "faith and morals"—or at least that seems implied even though the pope does not explicitly refer to the definition of Vatican I in remarks about the natural law.

This view is quite explicit in the encyclical *Humanae Vitae*, July 25, 1968, as well. In the usual section at the beginning of the encyclical dealing with the authority of the Church, Pope Paul writes:

No believer will deny that the teaching authority of the Church is competent to interpret even the natural moral law. It is, in fact, indisputable, as our predecessors have many times declared, that Jesus Christ, when communicating to Peter and to the Apostles His divine authority and sending them to teach all nations His commandments, constituted them as guardians and interpreters of all the moral law, not only, that is, of the law of the Gospel, but also of the natural law, which is also an expression of the will of God, the faithful fulfillment of which is equally necessary for salvation.[14]

Note that Pope Paul asserts that it is the *teaching* authority of the Church which embraces the natural law and not just its *pastoral* authority. The view of Pius XII has been modified.

The matter of authority of the hierarchy is touched upon also—but much more lightly—in the encyclical *Populorum Progressio* of March 26, 1967. In both encyclicals appeal is made to papal statements on a variety of issues dating from Pius IX in the case of *Humanae Vitae* and from Leo XIII in the case of *Populorum Progressio*.

The teaching, then, seems clear enough: The deposit of revelation has been given to the pope and the bishops who teach with an authority that is independent of the reasons they may give for their moral directives. This teaching authority derives from the authority of the Church to teach in matters of faith and morals and it extends to the whole field of morals, including the natural moral law.

II

In an article published on the centenary of the First Vatican Council's definition of papal infallibility, Karl Rahner considered some of the problems posed by the notion of a teaching authority that is authoritative but not infallible.[15]

In his 1970 discussion of the concept of infallibility, Rahner remarks, almost in passing at the end, in the context of the question whether there can be new infallible statements by the Church, that the Church has in fact hardly ever made such a new definition, not even at the Second Vatican Council or in *Humanae Vitae*, despite the fact that some of the questions being dealt with were of the greatest importance.[16] Rahner suggests that one of the reasons for this situation is the historical character of statements in moral theology and the dynamic and hence changing character of the reality (i.e., human nature) to which they point as normative.[17]

In another article published in 1970 Rahner addressed himself directly to the question of the noninfallible but authentic *magisterium*. The context of his remarks is instructive. The German bishops issued in 1967, after *Humanae Vitae*, a doctrinal statement[18] on the teaching authority and the teaching mission of the Church. Among the subjects considered was the possibility of dissent from "provisional"—i.e., the noninfallible but authentic statements of the *magisterium*—a dissent that the bishops recognized as a possibility, at least under some circumstances.

An anonymous critic of the bishops' position published and circulated a statement denying the possibility of such dissent because, he argued, the binding character of the statement of the *magisterium* is derived not from the arguments offered but from the authority of those who teach. Hence any dissent is an act of disobedience. The critic had obviously read Pius XII.

Rahner's article[19] is a reply and critique of this anonymous statement. He characterizes the position it defends as "fundamentally false." He finds it ironic that so vehement a defender of the teaching authority of bishops should make the teaching of the German bishops the object of his criticism. Granted that there can be and are thoroughly worthless reasons for rejecting the "provisional" teaching of the *magisterium*, Rahner insists, nevertheless, that under certain circumstances a Catholic Christian has the right and even the moral obligation to dissent from "provisional" teaching. This the critic of the German bishops will not concede.

In the first place, Rahner argues, it is not difficult to produce numerous examples of statements made by the *magisterium* which today are recognized as simply wrong. He offers examples from the decisions of the Pontifical Biblical Commission that have never been officially revoked and from statements that denounced proposals for the reform of the Holy Office or for the abolition of the Index of Forbidden Books as smacking of modernism. At other times the *magisterium* has held that polygenism was incompatible with a properly understood doctrine of original sin. Anybody who learned his theology more than fifteen years ago in a typical seminary could extend the list without difficulty. I think I need not illustrate further from such older questions as the taking of interest on loans[20] or the legitimacy of sexual relations for a married couple when they do not have at least the intention of procreation —which, take note, is quite a different question than the modern one of contraception. Clearly the *magisterium* has made statements that were simply wrong.

But Rahner's principal argument is the simple one that the Church has made statements which are recognized as being erroneous and that it would be impossible on the terms of the argument given by the bishops' critic ever to correct these errors if no one is permitted to disagree with them. Nor does Rahner believe it possible to dissent only privately, given the rapid communication everywhere of ideas today. Rahner is very conscious that such possible dissent can be abused. But it is his contention that the possibility of abuse does not destroy the legitimacy and even the necessity of dissenting from magisterial teaching that is clearly noninfallible, when the reasons for that dissent are solidly grounded. In short, the possibility of genuinely "provisional" utterances of the *magisterium* must be conceded, utterances that are in principle open to correction and even to falsification.

One might suspect at this point that a theologian like Rahner would reduce the Church to silence on any number of issues. Nothing could be further from the truth. The fact is that I know of no Catholic theologian who has struggled as persistently as Rahner to understand the meaning of a *magisterium* which is at one and same time both genuinely authoritative in a religious sense and genuinely open to correction.

Some of Rahner's most interesting work along these lines has been done in essays that he devoted to the Pastoral Constitution on the Church in the Modern World issued by Vatican II. The tone and content of the Pastoral Constitution are familiar: it is 23,335 words long in its Latin text, and it offers extensive comment and direction on a wide variety of familial, social, political and economic problems.

Rahner writes[21] that a pastoral constitution consists in directives of the Church that arise from the Church's charismatic and hence religious grasp of the present situation as her decisions in response to the charismatic call of God.[22] The need for such pastoral directives, which involve more than the preaching of explicit gospel imperatives and carry the Church into the world, arises from the necessity of action in the world by the Church.[23]

I do not wish to pursue the details of Rahner's extensive study of a truly *pastoral* constitution with its directives, other than to point out Rahner's insistence that there must be a genuinely *religious* dimension to the Church's interventions in the world, which he attributes to the charismatic work of the Spirit. Such directives have moral authority because they are in response to the call of God in the particular concrete circumstances of the time and place for which they are issued. Because of their historicity and their secular character, pastoral directives are not simple commands but summonses to creative freedom. Their function is therefore limited: to be critical vis-à-vis the world, since the Church has no secular function, and yet to be obligatory for the members of the Church, since they are responsive to what God calls for here and now. All this is Rahner's attempt to understand the truly religious character of the Pastoral Constitution and its several chapters of such directives. He is studying what the Church is actually doing. The same analysis might apply to a document like *Populorum Progressio*. The *style* of such documents is more *dialogical* than *authoritative*.

There is one other suggestion of Rahner's worth noting here. Writing on the encyclical *Humanae Vitae*, Rahner says:

It becomes clear in the encyclical itself that the real and primary reason for adhering to this position is the need that is felt to hold firm to the traditional teaching of Pius XI and Pius XII. This fact certainly carries a not inconsiderable theological weight, the more so since in individual moral questions a certain global "instinct" can be right even when it is incapable of being explicated to the utmost at the level of rational theory and speculation. Yet in view of the fact that *according to the encyclical itself* what is in question here is not simply a divine revelation of a moral norm, but rather a principle of the "natural law," it would have been desirable for the material grounds for holding the papal thesis to have been justified by more precise arguments.[24]

Rahner has invoked the notion of a moral instinct in other contexts that I cannot review here. Let it suffice to say that again he is trying to find a basis for the authority of magisterial pronouncements—even when the pronouncements themselves offer little argument beyond sheer authority. The notion of an instinct for what is morally right or an instinct for the truth of faith is grounded in Rahner's understanding of a collective consciousness in the Church community that holds the faith, even if only in a prereflective way.[25] I mention the matter here in support of my contention that few theologians have worked as diligently as Rahner to understand and support the work of the *magisterium*.

III

After this lengthy discussion of Rahner, let me turn more briefly to one more discussion of the *magisterium* and the natural law. I refer to the work of the Swiss Jesuit theologian, Jacob David.[26] I will omit David's discussion of the Church's use of natural law in developing modern social doctrine as well as his discussion of the historicity of natural law and the mutability of human nature. I will focus on his discussion of the *magisterium* and the natural law.

David recalls the statement of Vatican II that infallibility extends as far as the deposit of revelation which must be religiously guarded and faithfully expounded.[27] Since the natural law is not a revealed law, David concludes that the Church's authority in matters of natural law derives not from its teaching authority but from its pastoral authority. (Recall that Pius XII had discussed the competence of the Church in natural law matters under the heading of the pastoral office.) David is, of course, thinking of the whole body of social teaching that has been developed since Leo XIII. He does not deny that there are revealed elements in this teaching, but his point is that much of it is expressly derived from the natural law and not from revelation.[28] David does not find problematic the competence of the Church to reject interpretations of the natural law that are incompatible with revelation[29] and even to declare that a system of natural law is compatible with revelation, so long as it is not implied that only some single philosophical system is compatible with revelation. What he does find problematic is a *positive* affirmation of the *magisterium* that is based solely on the natural law and yet is regarded as obligatory. It does not follow, he says, that because a moral doctrine is compatible with revelation it becomes obligatory. Many teachings on the same subject might be equally compatible with revelation.[30] Citing the statement of the Pastoral Constitution (n. 36) on the autonomy of the profane sciences, David denies that there is any theologi-

cal basis for the *magisterium* making obligatory positive pronouncements, although he freely concedes that the Church has
the duty to defend the natural moral law. But its theological
warrant can only be the *negative* one that a course of conduct is
not compatible with revelation.

It is David's contention that the modern popes employed
the natural law as the basis for their dialogue between the
Church and society because all other means of influencing society had disappeared. And he does not question at all the legitimacy of using arguments from reason that were comprehensible
and even persuasive to the modern mind. But he asks to what
extent such statements are really theological and therefore obligatory.[31] In asking the question he concedes that revelation does
indeed contain some few revealed moral matters, for example,
the commandment of love, even of one's enemies, the nature of
marriage and its sacred character. David then reaches this conclusion:

> First of all it seems established that only those questions of
> natural law which touch upon revealed data pertain to the
> *doctrinal magisterium* of the Church and that to these
> alone Catholics are obliged to give an assent of faith. They
> are of great importance, but their number is small and
> their content remains very general. The other problems of
> natural law—and these are the problems one encounters
> most of the time in practice—pertain to the *pastoral* func-
> tion of the Church, to its function as the guardian of
> morals. The authority of the Church acts here as a guide
> and has only a disciplinary character. It has the power,
> clearly, thus to give teaching on these problems *when* the
> good of Christianity or that of humanity requires it and to
> the extent that they require it. But, in this matter the
> Church finds itself up to a certain point on the same level
> as "every other human authority which has the necessary
> qualifications."[32]

The concluding observation about others teaching the natural
law David attributes to Pius XII on the basis of a study made

by K. Hormann.[33] David is persuaded that his approach frees the Church from a lot of dead weight and opens the way to dialogue and discussion with the whole of humanity in seeking just, which is to say human, solutions to our planetary problems.[34] Please note that he is not attempting to reduce the Church or its leaders to silence.

IV

I will now touch briefly on several aspects of our problem that have been the subject of recent study.

A number of scholars have looked into the notion of *magisterium* itself. The notion of an authoritative *magisterium* in the sense in which that term has been used in recent Catholic documents is not older than the nineteenth century.[35] Scholars have pointed out that the notion of teaching, for example, is not univocal: there are many kinds of teachers and they function in a great variety of ways.[36] Gregory Baum, for example, taking the sociological studies of Max Weber as a point of departure, has tried to sketch the function of religion in providing the values and ideals upon which societies are built. The Church shows her values to society not just through speeches, encyclical letters of conciliar constitutions, but also by the way in which the Church herself acts. Baum and others have suggested that the proper style of Church teaching today may very well not be authoritative pronouncements that do not even attempt to offer arguments for their point of view.

Still other scholars have looked at the notion of "faith and morals" that the First Vatican Council defined as the area of competence for the *magisterium* of the Church.[37] These scholars have pointed out that the *mores* in the traditional phrase included, as recently as the Council of Trent, matters much broader than our English term "morals" might suggest. Such things as liturgical customs and other matters of Church discipline were understood as included in the *mores* by Trent. Yet no one claims that the Church makes irreformable pronouncements in these areas. The Belgian historian Roger Aubert was asked a few years ago what the Fathers of the First Vatican Council meant by the *mores* of their definition. Aubert replied that they meant the broad principles of moral theology.[38]

Still another question has to do with the whole notion of authoritative pronouncements on matters of right and wrong. The British moral philosopher Elizabeth Anscombe[39] has pointed out that if one tells a child to do something and the child asks why, it makes sense to answer, "Because I said so." But if one tells a student that the sum of the interior angles of a triangle is 180 degrees, and he asks why, it would be curious, not to say pointless, to reply, "Because I said so." Part of this consideration lies in the fact that it seems that an action done solely because someone told the agent to do it, without the agent's having made his own moral judgment about the moral rightness or wrongness of the action, does not seem to be a moral action at all. It seems necessary that the agent's own conscience be somehow engaged in the agent's doing a good action because it is judged by him to be good. This is not to suggest that each individual's conscience is all-sufficient or infallible or that one need not seek advice and direction in a great variety of matters. It means only that when the advice and direction and consultation have taken place, a moral agent must still make a moral decision that is his own. Such a decision may, of course, be wrong; but it does not seem possible simply to substitute the judgment and decision of another for one's own moral responsibilities.

V

Let me now try to summarize.

The Christian faith proclaimed in and by the Church implies both things that are to be believed and things that are to be done. Faith implies both *credenda* and *agenda*. Raymond Collins pointed out, in the article cited in chapter two, that in working out the norms of the Christian life the New Testament emphasized formal norms over material ones and borrowed freely from a variety of sources in developing material norms. The result was a pluralism of ethics even within the New Testament.[40]

It should be emphasized, I think, that this pluralism notwithstanding, teachers in the Church have given much practical advice and laid down numerous material norms for the Christian life. The community is the matrix within which the Christian learns what the Christian life requires, and it therefore has an indispensible role.

Catholic theologians today commonly affirm the duty of the Church to proclaim the Christian message and the moral values that it contains or clearly implies. The freedom and dignity of each human person before God is such a value and the constant theme of recent Church pronouncements, one of the latest being a statement of "Human Rights and Reconciliation" published by Pope Paul together with the 1974 Synod of Bishops.[41]

Catholic theologians like Karl Rahner and Jacob David also recognize that it is the duty of the Church to speak on specific moral issues. But what is increasingly under fire is a juridical notion of the *magisterium*, which invests the pronouncements of officeholders in the Church with an authority that is independent of the reasons for their pronouncements—even when the basis for the pronouncement is the natural law, which by definition is the product of reason in the tradition of St. Thomas. Peter Knauer, for one, has pointed to this absence of explanation as a key weakness of *Humanae Vitae*.[42]

It follows then that the emphasis falls increasingly on the need to proclaim the formal norms demanded by the Christian message. But when it comes to specific questions and material norms, theologians stress less juridical authority and more the critical and prophetic role of the Church. Karl Rahner, for one, has spoken of the "liberating modesty" with which the Church must confront the world.[43] And others, like Gregory Baum, have emphasized that formal teaching is by no means the only way in which the Church tells the world what it believes to be important.

All this, of course, has important implications for the field of medical ethics, including sterilization. No longer will it do simply to repeat "natural law" prohibitions in the form of officially imposed norms without the ethical argument that can elicit assent. Neither would it be faithful to the gospel to collapse into silence about the important values that are at stake in the discussion about sterilization and the broader argument over contraception. Other and more appropriate forms of teaching, including the crucial *praxis* of institutions sponsored by the

Church, will, I believe, play an increasing role.[44]

In the hospital and its activities the values proclaimed by the Church, the multiple areas of professional expertise represented by the hospital staff, and the claims of conscience of the hospital, the staff, and the patients come together. In the next chapter we turn to the hospital and its relationship to the Church and its officials.

Perhaps this chapter can conclude appropriately with a sobering reminder by the German bishops, in the 1967 doctrinal letter cited by Karl Rahner, on the subject of dissent from the noninfallible teachings of the papal and episcopal *magisterium*. The right, and even the duty, of a believer to dissent has been restated often since *Humanae Vitae* by theologians, historians, and canonists. The German bishops wrote:

> Anyone who believes that he can retain his own private opinion, and that he is already even now in possession of that better insight which the Church will achieve in the future must take stock of himself in an attitude of sober self-criticism, and ask himself before God and his own conscience whether he has the necessary breadth and depth of specialized theological knowledge to be able to deviate from the current teaching of the official Church in his private theory and practice. Such a case is in principle conceivable. But subjective presumptuousness and over-hasty opinionatedness will have to answer before the judgment of God.[45]

It is a sometimes uncomfortable fact of contemporary life in the Catholic Church that on more than one question about which the official teaching authority of the Church has spoken, not a few Catholics are risking just that judgment.

Notes

1. See Raymond Collins, "Scripture and the Christian Ethic," in *Proceedings of the Catholic Theological Society of America,* 29

(1974), pp. 215-41; Bernard-Dominique Dupuy, "The Constitutive Nature of Ethics in the Confession of the Christian Faith," *Concilium*, n. 51 (1970), 68-78; Joseph Fuchs, S.J., "Moral Theology and Dogmatic Theology," in *Human Values and Christian Morality*, trans. by M. H. Heelan, *et al.* (Dublin: Gill and Macmillan, 1970, pp. 148-77; Karl Rahner, *Theological Investigations*, trans. by David Bourke (New York: Seabury, 1974), XI, pp. 144-45; O. Semmelroth, "Orthodoxis und Orthopraxis. Zur wechselseitigen Begründung von Glaubenserkennen und Glaubenstun," *Geist und Leben*, 42 (1969), 359-73.

2. See Joseph Fuchs, S.J., "Origines d'une trilogie, ecclésiologique a l'époque rationaliste de la théologie," *Revue des sciences philosophiques et théologiques*, 53 (1969), 185-211; T. Howland Sanks, S.J., *Authority in the Church: A Study in Changing Paradigms*, AAR Dissertation Series, n. 2 (Missoula: Scholars Press, 1974); Yves Congar, *Tradition and Traditions* (New York: Macmillan, 1967), pp. 177-229, esp. pp. 183-221; Walter Kasper, *Die Lehre von der Tradition in der Römischen Schule (G. Perrone, C. Passaglia, C. Schrader)* (Freiburg: Herder, 1962).

3. DS 3074; Neuner-Roos, 388.

4. LG, n. 25.

5. *Ibid.*, DB 2113.

6. DV, n. 10.

7. The term "deposit of faith" has its roots in the New Testament. Cf., e.g., Jude, 3; I Tim. 1:3-4. See D. Maguire in n. 36 below.

8. See DV, nn. 2-6 and, e.g., Gabriel Moran, F.S.C., *The Theology of Revelation* (New York: Herder & Herder, 1966).

9. What follows is a summary of the allocutions *Si Diligis* of May 31, 1954, and *Magnificate Dominum Mecum* of November 2, 1954, *The Pope Speaks*, 1 (1954), 153-58 and 375-85.

10. TPS, p. 156.

11. TPS, pp. 380-81.

12. *Ibid.*, p. 381.

13. *Ibid.*, p. 382.

14. *Humanae Vitae*, n. 4. (Washington: USCC, 1968).

15. What follows is derived from "Disput um das kirchliche Lehramt: Zum problem nicht-unfehlbarer kirchlicher Lehrentscheidungen"; *Schriften zur Theologie*, X (Zurich: Benziger Verlag, 1972), pp. 324-37; "Zum Begriff der Unfehlbarkeit in der katholischen Theologie," *Schriften*, X, pp. 305-23; "Zur Enzyklika 'Humanae Vitae,' " *Schriften*, IX, pp. 276-301; *Theological Investigations*, XI, pp. 263-87; and *The Shape of the Church to Come*, trans. by Edward Quinn (New York: Seabury, 1974).

16. It should be noted that Rahner does occasionally refer to a moral command as a faith-statement, e.g., "Murder is a sin," in *The Christian of the Future* (New York: Herder and Herder, 1967), pp.

21-22; he refers to the gospel as a source of moral direction in *Investigations*, II, p. 100; *Schriften*, VIII, p. 641ff. and p. 670; IX, pp. 186 and 295; and in *The Dynamic Element in the Church* (New York: Herder and Herder, 1964), p. 91.

17. *Schriften*, X, p. 322.
18. Text in *Investigations*, XI, pp. 268-70.
19. "Disput . . ."
20. See John Noonan, *The Scholastic Analysis of Usury* (Cambridge: Harvard, 1957), p. 325 for the statement and excommunication by Alexander VII in 1666, and Noonan's comment on *Humanae Vitae*, in *The Birth Control Debate*, ed. by Robert G. Hoyt (Kansas City: *National Catholic Reporter*, 1968), pp. 181-84.
21. See "On the Theological Problems Entailed in a 'Pastoral Constitution,' " in *Investigations*, X, pp. 293-317.
22. *Ibid.*, pp. 311-12.
23. *Ibid.*, pp. 307-08.
24. *Investigations*, XI, p. 266.
25. *Investigations*, XI, p. 286. Rahner attaches an important role to the work of the *magisterium* in articulating the unreflective faith-consciousness.
26. What follows is taken from Jacob David, *Loi naturelle et autorité de l'Eglise* (Paris: Les Editions du Cerf, 1968) [German: *Das Naturrecht in Krise und Läuterung* (Cologne: Bachem, 1967)]. See also his "Kirche und Naturrecht: Versuch einer neuen Grenzziehung," *Orientierung*, 30 (1966), 129-33.
27. LG, n. 25.
28. David, *Loi naturelle*, p. 75.
29. *Ibid.*, p. 78.
30. *Ibid.*, p. 80.
31. *Ibid.*, p. 87.
32. *Ibid.*, pp. 100-101 (my translation).
33. K. Hörmann, "Die Zuständigkeit der Kirche für das Naturrecht nach der Lehre Pius XII," in *Naturordnung in Gesellschaft: Festschrift für J. Messner*, ed. by J. Höffner, A. Verdross and F. Vito (Innsbruck-Vienna-Munich, 1961), pp. 139-50.
34. David, *Loi naturelle*, p. 101.
35. See Note 2.
36. See Daniel Maguire, "Moral Absolutes and the Magisterium," in *Absolutes in Moral Theology?*, ed. by Charles E. Curran (Washington: Corpus, 1968), pp. 57-107; Gregory Baum, "Does Morality Call for the Church?", in *Proceedings of the CTSA*, 25 (1970), 159-73.
37. Maurice Bevenot, S.J., " 'Faith and Morals' in the Councils of Trent and Vatican I," *The Heythrop Journal*, 3 (1962), 15-30; Jacob David, S.J., "Glaube und Sitten: eine missverständliche Formel," *Orientierung*, 35 (1971), 32-34; Piet Fransen, " 'Geloof en

zeden': Notitie over een veelgebruikte formule," *Tijdschrift voor Theologie*, 9 (1966), 315-26; J. L. Murphy, *The Notion of Tradition in John Driedo* (Milwaukee, 1959), pp. 296-300.

38. Roger Aubert in *Infallibilité*, ed. by E. Castelli (Paris, 1961); Daniel Maguire, "Moral Inquiry and Religious Assent," in *Contraception, Authority and Dissent*, ed. by Charles E. Curran (New York: Herder & Herder, 1969), 127-48.

39. Elizabeth Anscombe, "Authority in Morals," in *Problems of Authority*, ed. by John M. Todd (Baltimore: Helicon, 1962), pp. 179-88. See also Franz Böckle, "Unfehlbare Normen?" in *Fehlbar: eine Bilanz*, ed. by Hans Küng (Zürich: Benziger, 1973), pp. 280-304.

40. See Note 1 above.

41. Text in *The Catholic Messenger*, Nov. 7, 1974.

42. Peter Knauer, S.J., "Überlegungen zur moraltheologischen Prinzipienlehre der Enzyklika 'Humanae Vitae,'" *Theologie und Philosophie*, 45 (1970), 60-74, at pp. 72-73.

43. Karl Rahner, "Church and World" in *Sacramentum Mundi*, I, pp. 346-57.

44. On the *magisterium* and morals see also Avery Dulles, S.J., "What Is *Magisterium*? Roles of Bishops and Theologians," *Origins*, 6, n. 6 (July 1, 1976), 81-88; Richard A. McCormick, S.J., "The Teaching Role of the *Magisterium* and of Theologians," *Proceedings of the Catholic Theological Society of America*, 24 (1969), 239-54, and "Notes on Moral Theology: Morality and the Competence of the *Magisterium*," *Theological Studies*, 30 (1969), 653-68. Yves Congar has recently published an important word study and historical analysis of the term *magisterium:* "Pour une histoire sémantique du terme 'Magisterium'," *Revue des sciences philosophiques et théologiques* 60 (January, 1976) 85-98 and "Bref historique des formes du 'Magistère' et de ses relations avec les docteurs," *Ibid.*, pp. 99-112.

45. In Karl Rahner, *Theological Investigations*, XI, p. 269.

4.
Sterilization in a
Catholic Hospital?

I

The relationship of Catholic hospitals to the Church has been the subject of considerable discussion in recent years. Not only have questions about the ethical code for Catholic hospitals been raised, but the increasing intrusion of government and third-party payers into the relationship of the hospital to its patients and into the operation of the hospital raises important questions about the autonomy of privately held, religiously sponsored health-care facilities.

The 1971 code of *Ethical and Religious Directives for Catholic Health Facilities*[1] describes the witness of the Catholic health facility "by fidelity to the Church's teachings while ministering to the good of the whole person." The total good of the patient, "which includes his higher spiritual as well as his bodily welfare," is so important a concern of the Catholic health facility "that if an institution could not fulfill its basic mission in this regard, it would have no justification for continuing its existence as a Catholic health facility." The Catholic health facilities exist because of the dedication of individuals "whose lives have been inspired by the Gospel and the teachings of the Catholic Church."

The link with the official teaching of the Church is fundamental: "Any facility identified as Catholic assumes with this identification the responsibility to reflect in its policies and practices the moral teachings of the Church under the guidance of the local bishop." Moreover: "The Catholic-sponsored health facility and its board of trustees, acting through its chief executive officer, further, carry an overriding responsibility in con-

71

science to prohibit those procedures which are morally and spiritually harmful." These are described in the code of ethical directives, and it follows that "any attempt to use a Catholic health facility for procedures contrary to these norms would indeed compromise the board and administration in its responsibility to seek and protect the total good of its patients, under the guidance of the Church." That guidance which deals with "the moral evaluation of new scientific developments and legitimately debated questions must be submitted to the teaching authority of the Church in the person of the local bishop, who has the ultimate responsibility for teaching Catholic doctrine."

In the current debate over the permissibility of sterilization, the letter to American bishops from the president of the National Conference of Catholic Bishops, Archbishop Joseph L. Bernardin of Cincinnati, on April 14, 1975, concluded that "Catholic hospitals, as a matter of institutional policy, may not authorize sterilization procedures for reasons other than those contained in the guidelines."

Again, the superordinate relationship of Church officers and their decisions to the hospital as organization or institution is taken for granted.

Underlying the letter of Archbishop Bernardin is the reply of the Sacred Congregation for the Doctrine of the Faith, dated March 13, 1975,[2] to the inquiries of the American bishops, made a year earlier, on the subject of therapeutic sterilization. After restating the papal *magisterium's* prohibition of sterilization as an intrinsic evil, the letter of the Congregation comments on the role of the hospital:

Any cooperation which involves the approval or consent of the hospitals to actions which are in themselves, that is, by their nature and condition, directed to a contraceptive end, namely, in order that the natural effects of sexual actions deliberately performed by the sterilized subject be impeded, is absolutely forbidden. For the official approbation of direct sterilization and, *a fortiori*, its management and execution in accord with hospital regulations, is a matter, which, in the objective order, is by its very nature (or intrinsically) evil. The Catholic hospital cannot cooperate with this for any reason. Any cooperation so supplied is totally unbecoming the mission entrusted to this type of institution and would be contrary to the necessary proclamation and defense of the moral order.[3]

The clear implication of this statement is that the Catholic hospital has a role in the proclamation and defense of the moral order. And again the bishops' questions and the Congregation's reply focus on the official or interorganizational relationship between the hospital and Church officials. It should be noted too that this is a relationship of the subordinate hospital to superordinate Church officials, as the very existence of the code, the bishops' questions and the Congregation's response make clear.

This interorganizational relationship of Church and hospital in the United States has usually taken the form of Church sponsorship of hospitals. The hospital is usually under the direction of a religious community or diocese, which in canon law forms a "moral person," and in civil law a corporation. The hospital is then usually incorporated separately, but with arrangements that give the sponsoring religious group decisive control through its control of the corporate membership, majority membership on the board of directors, or some other similar arrangement.[4] Thus the organizational relationship is strongly reinforced in the United States by legal and canonical arrangements that vest ownership and control of the hospital in the religious sponsor who is, in turn, tied by legal and canonical arrangements to the hierarchy of Church authority.

Traditionally, then, the relationship of the Church as organization to the hospital as organization has been a vertical one, with the hospital in a well-defined position of subordination to the sponsoring Church organization. Since the Church-sponsored hospital was a voluntary one, a good deal of homogeneity could be expected in the basic commitments and values held by the sponsoring religious group, the hospital administration, the physicians, nurses, staff, and even the patients. As a private institution, the hospital corporation was master in its own house, although the influence of the medical staff has always been great, and the medical profession was largely self-governing and self-regulating. The contributed services of the religious personnel helped the hospital to be financially self-sufficient. Although hospitals often had priest-chaplains, day-to-day intervention by bishops or other Church authorities was rare.

Sweeping changes both in the Church and in the general society have created quite a different situation for the Catholic health facility today.[5] Health insurance has created an interest of insurance carriers in the quality and cost of hospital care. Hospitals themselves have undertaken programs of accreditation that place heavy demands upon hospital resources. New technologies in the health-care field impose staggering expenses upon hospitals. Government intervention in the form of subsidies for the building of hospitals, provision of health care for the aged and other dependent segments of the population, and most recently health-care facilities planning has eroded the independence of the private health-care facility and places heavy strains on the vertical subordination of Church-sponsored hospitals to the Church hierarchy. Increasing pressures are exerted by other organizations, both public and private, for recognition of the interdependence of the private Church-sponsored hospital and other organizations in our complex society. Not only government agencies but private organizations, including consumer groups, demand an account from the hospital.

While it is true that many Catholic hospitals in the United States have for years served not only Catholics but have in fact been community facilities, it is also true that the renewal of the Catholic Church initiated by the Second Vatican Council has produced in the Church a rather new appraisal of the rights, convictions and values of persons who are not Catholics. The Council's documents on religious freedom and on the Church in the modern world represent important moves recognizing the *de facto* pluralism of the contemporary world and the inviolable rights of conscience of those who do not share Catholic convictions. Thus, at the same time that external pressures on the Catholic hospital urge the revision of the vertical model of relationships between the Catholic hospital and the constituencies that it serves—that indeed urge the recognition that there is a plurality of constituencies to which the Catholic hospital is accountable—the post-conciliar period has brought important modifications of the way in which Catholic Church organizations understand themselves and their relation to Church authorities and other organizations. The hospital under Church sponsorship which is *de facto* a community institution, in the sense that it serves the larger community, is staffed by members of that community who do not share at least some convictions of the Catholic Church, and is financed in significant and increasing measure by tax monies: such a hospital, even if its ownership and control are vested in a Church organization, cannot hope to escape accountability to increasingly various constituencies.

This changing situation suggests two areas in which the relationship of the Church and the hospital needs exploration. The first is at the level of interaction between two organizations, the health-care facility and the Church. But more specifically I wish to inquire into the particular role of theology and theological positions as these relate to the hospital. The relation of the hospital as organization to the Church and theology is reciprocal: the way in which theology conceptualizes the hospital and its functioning will have important consequences for the posing and solving of theological problems. Then it will be possible to discuss the policy of the hospital toward sterilization.

II

The modern general hospital is a complex organization.[6] Within the hospital, physicians skilled in a variety of medical specialties collaborate with nurses also skilled in various specialties and with a great number of technicians and other health-care professionals. The work of the health-care professionals is supported by other staff members who provide everything from bookkeeping to food service to maintenance. The administration manages the hospital to facilitate their collaboration. While hospitals vary greatly in size, services and complexity, even smaller hospitals provide an increasing array of services through their physicians and support staff.

For all their complexity, hospitals are not organized along vertical bureaucratic lines, with clear lines of subordination and superordination throughout. A hospital bears little resemblance to a military organization, with its rigid vertical relationships of rank and its multiple mechanisms, including force, if need be, to maintain the authority of superiors over their subordinates.

Perhaps the most obvious example of the unusual organizational pattern of the hospital is the relationship of the staff physician to the hospital. The physician brings to his work his own professional competence, certified by his graduation from an accredited medical school and his license granted by the state. Nothing in the professional competence of the hospital board or the hospital administration gives to either the power to command the professional decisions of the physician as he cares for his patients in the hospital. The physician (with some exceptions) is not an employee of the hospital but an independent contractor providing care to his patients in the hospital under conditions spelled out in the contract that admitted the physician to the hospital staff. Nurses and other professionals are typically employed by the hospital.

The result of this arrangement is a double line of authority in the hospital: one based on the professional competence of the physician, which the hospital cannot command, and the other based on the administrative and managerial responsibilities of the hospital corporation itself. For this reason the hospital as an organization resembles more a university than a government bureaucracy or a business enterprise, since relationships within the hospital organization have multiple and potentially conflicting grounds. The large modern hospital has reached such a degree of complexity that writers on organizational theory can speak of the hospital as a complex system made up of a large number of subsystems, each of which is itself a complex organizational system.

In a complex organization what is it that keeps large numbers of persons working together to achieve the purposes of the organization? Highly structured, closed organizations, say a prison or a monastery, achieve their purposes either by imposing or requiring acceptance of controls over every aspect of the life of persons within the organization and of a system of sanctions for deviation from the required pattern of behavior.

Other kinds of organizations, say a business enterprise, can provide monetary rewards, executive prestige, and job security for those in the organization who promote its purposes. Such enterprises have economic sanctions in particular to encourage or even compel compliance with organizational purposes.

It is apparent that the more an organization depends upon the professional skills of a large variety of persons to achieve its organizational purpose the less successful will be the techniques of motivation and cooperation that suffice in other kinds of organized undertakings. In every organization there is needed some degree of shared purpose, unless the organization can be made to succeed by sheer force. That perhaps is enough for the prison or at times for the military, but it will hardly do when the cooperation of skilled professionals is needed to provide high quality health care. In fact the *kind* of cooperation is different too, since what is needed from the professional is not simply physical presence or pouting compliance but the use of professional skills and the making of professional judgments that the hospital organization *per se* cannot use or make. More important than coercion in the complex organization which is the modern hospital is the power of shared ideas and values.

The glue that holds organizations together and makes them function effectively is often named "ideology" in the literature of organizational theory. A theologian may be excused for being a trifle uncomfortable with such an easily pejorative term, but I want to contend here that in the existence and operation of the Catholic hospital theology has a vital *ideological* role. What makes the religiously sponsored hospital what it is, what provides the *raison d'être* for the establishment and operation of hospitals by religious groups, is a theology. It is because Catholic Christians experience a summons to *diakonia*,[7] to the service of others, that they have banded together to operate hospitals. In giving service to the sick and to the dying, Catholic Christians, and other Christian groups that have organized and operate hospitals, bear witness to their Christian discipleship and to their obedience to Christ's demand for *agape*, love. Such motivation created the first hospitals for the care of the sick and dying as well as other institutions for the care of orphans and other dependent children and adults in the West, and in the United States it has created an impressive network of hospitals of all sorts.[8]

This public witness is an important form of teaching by the Church through the religious sponsor of the hospital. It is not so much teaching on a master/disciple model in which it can be taken for granted that the master is the depository of wisdom that is to be transmitted to the disciple, but rather teaching on a dialogic model in which the meanings and values that inform the religious sponsorship of the hospital interact with the diverse definitions and requirements of quality health care and with the needs and wants of both the hospital staff and the public. The hospital as such, and even more clearly the religious sponsor, has no qualifications to command the judgments of the medical professionals. A hospital cannot teach by *fiat*.[8a]

If then, religious convictions—theological ideas—have helped to create religiously sponsored hospitals, those same convictions have provided the ideology that made it possible for many persons with a variety of professional expertise to collaborate in providing quality health care. In an era when at least some basic Christian beliefs were widely accepted in American society, a Catholic hospital could expect to find wide agreement among the religious sponsor, physicians, professional staff, support staff, the administrators and the public being served about the purposes and functions of a community hospital. The presence of men and women religious, especially sisters, in the hospitals gave visible witness to the religious concern of the sponsoring group.

It is notoriously difficult to set out in concrete detail the implications of such a governing ideology for the day-to-day operation of an organization. Catholic hospitals have had a code of ethical directives for many years that spelled out certain specific concerns, and Catholic theologians did pioneering work in the field of medical ethics, applying the principles and techniques of moral theology to the solution of medical-ethical problems. Catholic hospitals enjoyed a reputation for loving care, especially for the seriously ill and the dying. The hospitals were better prepared than others, perhaps, to resist a purely technological approach to hospital care and to provide for the personal and religious needs of their patients through the staff sisters, the hospital chaplain and, more recently, through programs of pastoral care.[9]

Nevertheless, it is true that forging a link between the governing ideology of an organization and particular operational directives of an ethical code is no easy matter. In our own day, when the convictions of the religious sponsor may well not be shared by many on the staff or by many of the patients, the problems of the Catholic hospital in maintaining its sense of religious identity are complicated indeed. Is it possible today so to articulate the theological concerns that underlie the establishment and operation of a religiously sponsored hospital that the religious convictions of the sponsor can function as the "ideology," i.e., "the organizational values and shared norms, attitudes and mutual understanding, which can serve to provide a common universe of discourse for the different groups and members, and to socialize and bind the members securely into the system . . ."?[10] It is this ideology, the shared meanings, values and norms, that integrate the disparate elements of the organization into an articulated and functioning whole.

The difficulties of such a task ought not to be underestimated. It is easier to ask the various elements of the hospital organization to collaborate in providing quality health care for patients, a task that can be and is carried on in government health-care facilities throughout the U.S. without any explicit commitment to religious meanings and values. Dr. Edmund D. Pellegrino has argued that there is no generally accepted theory of values for the health of the nation against which priorities can be set, individual programs evaluated,[11] and resources allocated. If that is true of the social system of health-care delivery as a whole, it is equally true of the diverse communities served by the Catholic hospitals of the country. The values of the health-care system as a whole in American society will, presumably, be secular values, whatever their implicit religious underpinnings. The task of the religious organization which must define and articulate the meanings and values that make the religiously sponsored hospital distinctive and worth preserving in the national health-care delivery system taking shape under the compulsion of federal and state health-care planning legislation is clearly an urgent one—and one that is only getting underway. The stakes are very high: the very existence of the religiously sponsored private hospital.

Dr. Pellegrino has recently suggested that the Catholic hospital is informed by the concept of the Mystical Body:

> In this view, the Catholic hospital, those who administer and staff it, and the patients it serves are all bound together in a special community. They are united in the Mystical Body in a spiritual way proceeding from God and from Christ. The whole, as Congar asserts, is a "vast sacrament." What Catholic hospitals do for those they serve, they therefore do in a special way which unites man's earthly and spiritual destiny, linking server and served by a unique bond impossible to conceive in a secular institution, no matter how "concerned" it may be.[12]

Moreover the Catholic hospital has a view of what man is and of the place of sickness and suffering in human life. It is from these fundamental beliefs, Pellegrino contends, that the unique ethical perspectives of the Catholic hospital are derived. Pellegrino concedes that the ethical code is controversial:

> Nonetheless, what is unique to the Catholic hospital is that it does stand for a moral code that unites the religious, existential, and the moral dimensions of man's life. Catholic hospitals' positions on abortion, euthanasia, the rights of the fetus, the right to die with dignity, the right to disclosure, the right to refuse to undergo procedures, the right to privacy—indeed, all the current medical-moral dilemmas— must be derived and structured from the idea of the Church and the idea of man which grow out of revelation and tradition. They are the prelogical foundations which give authenticity to a body of principles if they are properly to be called Catholic.[13]

Granted that Pellegrino is correct in saying that convictions about the nature of the human and religious community and the nature of mankind and the role of illness and death must provide the governing meanings and values that integrate the diverse operations of the Catholic hospital, there remains the problem of mediating the lofty principle through ethical reflection to the level of practical action. Pellegrino concedes the difficulty of the task:

> This authenticity cannot reside simply in strict adherence to the juridical content of a code of ethics. Such a misconception leads only to pharisaism. True authenticity derives only from adherence to the spirit of the Mystical Body and Christian humanism. When that spirit informs every action, then a hospital is Catholic in the sense we have defined it.[14]

Dr. Pellegrino's considerations are an attempt at defining the identity of the Catholic hospital. More such efforts are needed.[14a]

III

The Catholic hospital is bound to the Church by bonds that are in part legal and canonical and in part doctrinal and moral. The issue of sterilization and the stance of the hospitals toward it is then paradigmatic of the situation of a Catholic institution in American society which is bearing witness to its own religious faith by providing a service to a very diverse public at a time when the Vatican Council has affirmed the right of religious freedom.

The hospital is a complex organization in which a large number of highly trained persons collaborate to provide health care to patients. The moralist would say that the hospital corporation and the various professionals and other staff are "cooperating" in the enterprise of giving health care. In a traditional Catholic moral perspective, and in the approach to judgments of the goodness or evil of actions outlined in chapter two, there is little problem in qualifying this sort of cooperation as a clear moral good. Whatever the ontic or premoral evils, including

pain, great expense and even the risk of death, which are involved in providing health care, most procedures are not morally problematic. The good being sought outweighs the premoral
evils.

But sterilization is one procedure that is forbidden by the
code of ethical directives, and the ban has been restated by the
Congregation for the Doctrine of the Faith. Can a Catholic hospital cooperate in providing sterilizations? And if it can, under
what circumstances, and with what rationale can it do so?

The recent reply of the Congregation for the Doctrine of
the Faith to the National Conference of Catholic Bishops rejects any action on the part of the hospital that implies approval
of sterilization, including "its management and execution in accord with hospital regulations."

But the Congregation does recall traditional doctrine about
"material cooperation" which is permitted under circumstances
that traditional moral theology has developed.[15] We turn briefly
to the traditional teaching on "material cooperation."

Given the idea of intrinsically evil acts that I described in
chapter two, the traditional teaching on material cooperation
attempted to find a way of neither *doing* evil or *intending* evil
when it was judged not possible to avoid all involvement with
evil.

I have already pointed out that in a complex organization
like a hospital cooperation in the actions of others is an absolute necessity. In a traditional notion of cooperation there was
no problem in this since the actions with which various persons
in the hospital and the hospital corporation itself cooperated
were seen to be morally good ones that contributed in one way
or another to the health of the patients. There could be a moral
problem about cooperation only when cooperation in the evil
actions of another was in question. Most textbook examples of
cooperation dealt with actions of individuals; one rarely saw any
discussion of the hospital corporation itself as a cooperator.

The contemporary authors who insist on an element of
ontic evil in every human action do not, of course, accept the
relatively uncomplicated view of moral reality presented by traditional textbooks. For the contemporary writers, each human

action is one with multiple effects, and even the best is shad-owed by ontic evil. Therefore cooperation with evil is not the exceptional thing envisioned by the textbooks, but the stuff of daily living. In sharing the world with other human beings whose actions are also shadowed by evil, we become coopera-tors in evil simply by co-existing in a world that is not wholly good.

The textbook tradition saw things more simply.[16] In deal-ing with cooperation in evil it forbade *doing* what is evil, i.e., actions which the tradition defined as "intrinsically evil," a cat-egory that the recent Roman document also uses. The tradition saw some actions as intrinsically evil, others as intrinsically good, but still others as morally indifferent. Aquinas' example of this latter category includes "picking up a stick from the ground."[17]

The tradition determined the moral goodness or evil of a concrete action by examining the object (i.e., the action itself as defined morally), the intention of the agent, and the circum-stances. Cooperation in the evil acts of another was of course forbidden, if the action to be performed was intrinsically evil. But if the action were good or at least indifferent, then coopera-tion might be possible without the agent's committing a moral fault. Turning then to the intention of the agent, the tradition held that the agent could not intend the evil in which the agent was somehow cooperating. How might that be possible? The tradition invoked the principle of double effect. One could per-form an action that was at least morally indifferent; one could foresee that from the performance of that act there would result an evil effect—the evil acts of another—but also a good effect, which alone could be directly intended by the agent. The evil ef-fect, though foreseen, had to be only indirect and outside the agent's intention. And as with any invocation of the principle of double effect, there had to be a proportion between the good ef-fect one foresaw and intended and the evil effect one foresaw but did not intend. The judgment of proportion was obviously the crux of the matter.

Here again the example of the war in Vietnam may be helpful. Once the judgment had been made that there was no

proportion between the goods being sought in Vietnam and the
havoc being wrought by the war, then even the principle of
double effect could no longer justify the carrying on of war there
or cooperation with the war. That moral judgment created problems of conscience for many Americans: from those who saw
their taxes being used to do what they judged to be evil to
draftees and those whose work was much more directly linked
to the war.

Catholic hospitals have been faced with problems of cooperation in a number of instances in which courts have ordered the
hospital to permit a physician to perform a tubal ligation, even
though the procedure was prohibited on religious grounds by
the hospital's code of ethics.[18] The procedures have been performed, presumably on the judgment that the evils that might
be visited upon a hospital which defied the federal courts outweighed the evil of sterilization itself. Since the hospital
explicitly rejected the sterilization procedure, its cooperation
was purely material, i.e., it yielded to the command of the court
and allowed its facilities to be used for the procedure (an action
that by traditional standards would be judged morally indifferent), although it well knew that the staff physician and the patient who had sought the court order would use the facilities for
purposes that the hospital did not approve. The sterilization itself was therefore (in the traditional analysis) not intended by
the hospital; what the hospital intended was only the use of its
facilities by a qualified physician in order to comply with the
court injunction. That obedience to the injunction offered the
occasion for the procedure of which the hospital did not approve was the factor that had to be judged: was the good which
the hospital sought (compliance with the injunction and the
avoidance of both the penalties for contempt of court and the
monetary damages that the plaintiffs also were seeking) propor-
tionately countervailing to the evil of the sterilization procedure
and the violence done to the hospital's convictions formulated in
the code of ethics? The judgment clearly was that there was an
acceptable proportion between those evils and the goods being
sought. But in the traditional analysis the hospital *did* no evil (it
performed acts that were morally indifferent) and it *intended* no

evil (it intended only obedience to the court order and avoidance of the penalties that would have followed defiance).

The traditional view would the more easily reach the decision that material cooperation was justified in the instance cited, since it would hold that the cooperation of the hospital is remote rather than proximate, i.e., the sterilization is not performed by the hospital corporation or its agents but by an independent contractor, the physician, and his immediate assistants. Legally,[19] nurses and other assistants to a physician in surgery are regarded as "borrowed servants" under the control of the physician rather than the hospital, even though they are hospital employees. This legal distinction reinforces the verdict of moralists who hold that the involvement of the hospital in court-ordered sterilizations is neither immediate nor proximate.

The meaning of the terms "necessary" and "free" cooperation is not altogether clear, in spite of the fact that the terms are used by the Congregation in its 1975 reply and also in a 1936 reply of the Holy Office on sterilization. Generally, authors use the term "necessary cooperation" to describe supportive actions without which an evil act could not be performed. Obviously such intimate cooperation with evil requires weighty justification. To describe other cooperative acts as "free" does not seem particularly apt, and even the alternative formulation "contingent cooperation" is not very helpful. The situation of a hospital under court order might, however, be properly described as that of a "necessary cooperator." The harm that might come to such a necessary cooperator is one factor that must be weighed in making the decision about whether or not to cooperate. Authors have held, for instance, that acts that are evil *per se*, e.g., blasphemy or idol worship, can never be performed no matter what the penalty for refusing. On the other hand, actions that are evil *ex defectu juris* or out of danger of sinning can be weighed against the harm that would result from a refusal to perform them. When the resulting harm assumes major proportions for the prospective agent, the defect of right or danger of sinning can yield to the overriding right of the cooperator to be free of the harm.[20] Needless to say, such acts remain evil for the principal agent. Zalba stresses this point in order to argue that in extraordinary circumstances, cooperation that is immediate, proximate and necessary to the performance of the evil act can be justified. Within the framework of the traditional analysis of cooperation, it is useful to draw attention to Zalba's opinion, which indicates the lengths to which a respected moralist is willing to go with cooperation in truly serious circumstances.

For Knauer, Schüller, Fuchs, Janssens, McCormick and others, the problem of cooperation is only another instance in which the judgment must be made whether the goods being sought are proportionate to the ontic evil institutional cooperation with sterilization would bring. Their analysis requires some redefinition of terms like "intrinsic evil," "direct" and "indirect" effects, etc. It also brings to the fore the particular problems of institutional cooperation.

This lengthy discussion of cooperation thus raises another question: the role of a corporation as a moral agent. The question arises because most of the examples in traditional moral theology assume that the moral agent is an individual. Most of the examples given in traditional books dealing with cooperation deal with the cooperation of one individual with another. But the question should be asked: Does a corporation as such function as a moral agent? And how does a corporation as such act?

The history of corporation law is instructive here.[21] Older corporation law held that corporations as such were incapable of committing torts or of violating the criminal law. The reasoning was that the corporation was a creature of the state, so that unlawful acts of corporate agents were *ultra vires*. Moreover, corporate entities were considered incapable of the criminal intent that is needed for violation of the criminal law.

Modern corporation law holds that corporations are capable of tortious acts and of violation of the criminal law. I need only mention unlawful campaign contributions revealed and prosecuted in the course of the Watergate investigations as examples of criminal violations of the law by corporations and their managers.

Canon law does not deal with moral persons in its section on crimes, apparently on the view that such acts are clearly *ultra vires*.

The moral obligations of corporate entities have played some role in the social ethics developed in the Catholic Church since the time of Leo XIII. For example, the moral obligations of business enterprises, with regard to the right of labor to organize (into other corporate entities), pricing policies, responsibility in the use of natural resources have been discussed in textbooks of social ethics.[22] More recently there has been developing a growing literature on the multinational corporation and the social obligations of corporate investors.[23] In every case it is assumed that corporate entities are moral agents with rights and responsibilities. Yet the typical moral theology textbook gave no attention to corporations as moral agents and the problems peculiar to their actions.

It does not seem necessary to argue here that corporations, whether business enterprises or nonprofit corporations like schools and hospitals, are indeed moral agents. A more useful question is: How does a corporation perform a moral act? The answer to that question is that corporations must make moral decisions in the same way that corporations make any kind of decision, i.e., through the action of the corporate board or of corporate managers invested with authority by board action to act on the corporation's behalf. It is my judgment that actions of corporate employees, which may well be actions of the corporation in the sense that the corporation is liable for the tortious actions of employees under the doctrine of *respondeat superior*, are corporate actions in the moral sense only negatively, i.e., insofar as the corporation has an affirmative duty through its managers to direct and supervise the actions of its employees and agents so as to avoid harm to others. But the negligent acts of an employee, even if the corporation is liable for their consequences, do not reflect a corporate moral decision in the absence of action or the abdication of its fiduciary responsibilities by the corporate board.

The need for action by the board or by someone holding authority from the corporate board is important, it seems to me, for a practical understanding of what is implied by "material cooperation." The recent Roman response on sterilization forbids approval of sterilization and *a fortiori* its management and execution in accord with hospital regulations.[24] But in the following paragraph the document goes on to discuss using "with utmost prudence" the traditional doctrine of material cooperation. How then is the hospital to employ the traditional doctrine of material cooperation and to explain its actions if the management of sterilization procedures is intrinsically evil—and that even more strongly than consent to the procedures?

It seems to me that it is mistaken to suppose that a corporation can somehow perform any act, even one of material cooperation with acts of which it does not approve, without an action by its board. In most cases, especially in the United States, where requests for sterilization are not an extraordinary occurrence, that will mean the establishment of a corporate policy on sterilization, even if the policy does no more than spell out the reasons and conditions under which a specific hospital will cooperate with a procedure that it disapproves on moral grounds. Some mechanics, a committee, for example, must be established to handle requests. The management of sterilization by the establishment of a corporate policy seems to me to be unavoidable; it need not imply moral approval at all. In the present legal climate a corporate policy which is or even appears to be capricious, or simply is left to the discretion of an administrator, might well invite suit by a staff physician and/or a patient. That would especially be the case in communities in which the Catholic hospital is, at least *de facto*, the community health facility.

It is of interest to recall that some Canadian hospital policies on sterilization, which have been drawn up as Catholic hospitals are made a part of provincial health-care delivery systems in that country, cast the hospital's role explicitly into the framework of cooperation[25] and set out the conditions under which the institution will cooperate in a sterilization procedure. The policy statements are not explicit in rejecting sterilization on moral grounds, nor do they set out at length reasons for believing that material cooperation is permissible. In at least some cases in Canada the judgment clearly was that sterilization is not an evil in every case so that the problem was not seen precisely as one of cooperating in evil; the hospital saw the sterilization as a good under some circumstances.[26]

In the American context and within the situation created

by the Roman response, it seems to me that hospitals which make the judgment that they must do some sterilizations in order to provide the health care demanded by the communities they and their staff physicians serve must continue to have policies stating clearly the situations in which they will cooperate to provide sterilization procedures, even though they regard the procedure as illicit. A policy of *laissez-faire*, of looking the other way, or of attempting to deal with problems on a case-by-case basis will hardly satisfy the medical staff and the communities that are served by Catholic hospitals, especially given the pluralism of views on sterilization conscientiously held by both medical professionals and the public. Nonpolicies and subterfuges can only lead to the discrediting of the Church's moral leadership and to potentially serious legal problems, since the alternative to an established policy will certainly be at least the appearance of arbitrariness.

The practical steps to be taken will therefore differ little whether one holds that sterilization is an intrinsically evil act and then follows the traditional doctrine of material cooperation, or whether one takes the view that a moral judgment can be made about sterilization only when the ontic evils it brings with it for the patient, for the hospital and for the common good can be weighed against the goods being sought. A corporation must have a corporate policy, and it can formulate one only when its corporate board and managers have taken various dimensions of the problem into consideration and formulated a hospital policy. Needless to say, diverse local circumstances can and will lead to diverse policies. It will be no surprise that the Catholic hospital which is the *de facto* community health facility for a large area or which is located in a part of the country in which its clientele is largely not Catholic may well arrive at a different policy than a Catholic hospital serving a Catholic clientele in a metropolitan area where other health facilities are available. Such diverse policies will witness not only to the diversity of views on the morality of sterilization, but more significantly to the variety of factors that must be taken into consideration in making a judgment about a concrete policy at a concrete place and time.

To conclude this chapter, I must anticipate an objection. If

Catholic hospitals adopt policies stating conditions under which they will cooperate in sterilizations in spite of the recent restatement of the papal *magisterium's* moral disapproval, is not the door opened to exactly the same course of action regarding abortion?

I have argued that there can be no escape from the responsibility of making moral judgments. Invoking a rule is not enough. The factors to be weighed must again be placed in the balance and a judgment made whether a proportion exists between the evil of abortion and whatever goods would be sought by permitting an abortion or at least cooperating materially with the procedure.

It is my judgment that the ontic evil of destroying human life, even unborn human life, is so serious that it is hard to imagine what countervailing value other than human life itself could justify it. Other values hardly seem proportionate to the evil of destroying innocent human life. Such a judgment might indeed be possible in cases in which abortion was truly demanded to save the life of a mother. But *it does not follow* that Catholic hospitals should adopt that position, even if there were no problems with canonical penalties. In the present American context, the ability of religiously sponsored hospitals to control their own ethical affairs in accordance with their religious convictions is threatened from several sides: not only by the orders of courts but by health-care planning agencies and third-party payers.

Therefore, important questions of social policy must also be taken into consideration in developing an institutional judgment regarding abortion and cooperation in the performance of abortion. I would find it difficult to justify even material cooperation with abortion by a Catholic hospital at the present time (except perhaps in the case where a woman's life could not otherwise be saved) for several reasons. First of all I believe that such cooperation would be tantamount to forfeiting the Catholic hospital's claim to control its ethical affairs. I assume that abortion is very rarely an emergency procedure and that alternatives are generally available in situations that threaten the life of a mother—though part of the witness of Catholic institutions must be to provide alternatives. Moreover, I find it difficult to judge that cooperation with abortion could be anything but scandalous—in the strong theological sense that even apparent capitulation by Church-sponsored institutions to abortion would lead others to sin. The sin is not simply loss of respect for innocent human life but a growing willingness to find in abortion a convenient solution to a pregnancy unwanted for any reason at all. In the present climate, there is an urgent need for a clear and prophetic No to abortion on demand from the Church and institutions that share its convictions.

My point then is that I regard the evils which would accompany an institutional policy of cooperation with abortion in Catholic hospitals as out of proportion to any good that such policies could realize. The situation with sterilization I judge to be different, and I believe that the practice of Catholic hospitals in recent years supports my conviction of a difference in the two questions. Because the goods and evils at stake are different, in my judgment cooperation with sterilization can be permitted while abortion must be resolutely rejected.

Notes

1. Washington: The United States Catholic Conference, 1971. The citations are from the preamble. Among the critiques of the Code, see Richard A. McCormick, S.J., "Not What Catholic Hospitals Ordered," *America*, 125 (1971), 510-13; and the exchange: Eugene F. Diamond, M.D., "A Physician Views the Directives," *Hospital Progress*, 53, n. 11 (November, 1972), 57-60; and Warren T. Reich and Richard A. McCormick, S.J., "Theologians View the Directives," *Hospital Progress*, 53, n. 12 (December, 1972), 50-54+68. The discussion continued in 54, n. 2 (February, 1973), 70-76. Much of *Chicago Studies*, 11, n. 3 (Fall, 1972) is devoted to a discussion of the code, with articles by Andre Helligers, M.D., Warren T. Reich, Richard A. McCormick, S.J., and Thomas O'Donnell, S.J. In addition, see the report of a committee of the Catholic Theological Society of America cited in note 5.
2. Prot. 2027/69. The document was distributed to the bishops with a cover letter from Bishop James S. Rausch, General Secretary of the NCCB, dated December 4, 1975. Text of the Roman response

in *Origins*, 6, n. 3 (June 10, 1976), 33-35. See also Kevin O'Rourke, "An Analysis of the Church's Teaching on Sterilization," *Hospital Progress*, 57, n. 5 (May, 1976), 68-75+80. Richard A. McCormick, S.J. has published a critical comment, "Sterilization and Theological Method," *Theological Studies*, 37 (1976), 471-77.

3. N. 3, in *Origins*, p. 35. The Latin reads: Quaevis eorum cooperatio institutionaliter adprobata vel admissa ad actiones ex seipsis (hoc est, ex natura et conditione ipsarum) in finem contraceptivum ordinatas, nimirum, ut impediantur effectus connaturales actuum sexualium a subiecto sterilizato deliberate admissorum, est absolute interdicta. Nam officialis approbatio sterilizationis directae, et a fortiori eiusdem secundum statuta nosocomii regulatio et executio, est res in ordine obiectivo indole sua seu intrinsice mala, ad quam hospitale catholicum nulla ratione potest cooperari. Quaevis cooperatio sic praestita omnino dedeceret missionem huiusmodi institutionibus concreditam, essetque contraria necessariae proclamationi et defensioni ordinis moralis.

4. See Adam J. Maida, JCL, JD, *Ownership Control and Sponsorship of Catholic Institutions* (Harrisburg: The Pennsylvania Catholic Conference, 1975); James A. Hamilton, *Patterns of Hospital Ownership and Control* (Minneapolis: University of Minnesota Press, 1961), pp. 89-102. Some alternative schemes of ownership for Catholic hospitals are suggested by Edmund D. Pellegrino, M.D., "The Catholic Hospital: Options for Survival," *Hospital Progress*, 56 (1975), 42-52.

5. For what follows, see, for example, the "Report of the Commission on the Ethical and Religious Directives for Catholic Hospitals of the Catholic Theological Society of America," *Linacre Quarterly*, 39 (1972), 2-24; the *CTSA Proceedings*, 27 (1972), 41-69; *Hospital Progress*, 54, n. 2 (February, 1973), 44-56. See also Donald J. Keefe, S.J., "A Review and Critique of the CTSA Report," in the same issue, pp. 57-69. See also Richard A. McCormick, S.J., "The New Directives and Institutional Medico-Moral Responsibility," in *Chicago Studies*, 11 (1972), 305-14, on the shift away from paternalism in medicine. I regard the shift from paternalism to consumerism in medicine as an important component of the contemporary situation for the Catholic hospital.

6. For the following section see Amitai Etzioni, *Comparative Analysis of Complex Organizations* (Glencoe: The Free Press, 1961); A. Etzioni, *Modern Organizations* (Englewood Cliffs: Prentice-Hall, 1964); A. Etzioni (ed.), *Complex Organizations: A Sociological Reader* (New York: Holt, Rinehart & Winston, 1966); Robert K. Merton, *Social Theory and Social Structure*, rev. ed. (New York: The Free Press, 1957); Talcott Parsons, *Structure and Process in Modern Societies* (Glencoe: The Free Press, 1960); T. Parsons,

The System of Modern Societies (Englewood Cliffs: Prentice-Hall, 1971); *Organization Research in Health Institutions* (Ann Arbor: The Institute for Social Research, University of Michigan, 1972), ed. by Basil S. Georgopoulos; *Hospital Organization and Management: A Book of Readings*, ed. by Jonathan S. Rakich (St. Louis, The Catholic Hospital Association, 1972). See also Robert J. Mulvaney, "Institutional Commitment," in *Educational Theory*, 21 (1971), 444-54. Although Mulvaney deals with the university context, his comments on the appropriateness of high-level commitments by the institution and the distinction he draws between the institution and the community seem to me applicable to the hospital situation too.

7. See for example, Hans Küng, *The Church*, trans. by Ray and Rosaleen Ockenden (New York: Sheed & Ward, 1967), pp. 388-444, and the chapter on "The Church as Servant" in Avery Dulles, S.J., *Models of the Church* (Garden City: Doubleday, 1974), pp. 83-96.

8. For a historical perspective on the involvement of the Christian Church in hospitals and health care, see Mary Risley, *House of Healing: The Story of the Hospital* (Garden City: Doubleday, 1961).

8a. See the discussion in chapter three.

9. See E. Pellegrino, "The Catholic Hospital."

10. Basil S. Georgopoulos, "The Hospital as an Organization and Problem-Solving System," in B. S. Georgopoulos (ed.), *Organization Research*, pp. 9-48, citation at p. 29.

11. Edmund D. Pellegrino, M.D., "The Changing Matrix of Clinical Decision-Making in the Hospital," in B. S. Georgopoulos (ed.), *Organization Research*, pp. 301-28, citation at p. 323.

12. E. Pellegrino, "The Catholic Hospital," p. 45.

13. *Ibid.*, p. 46.

14. *Ibid.*, p. 46.

14a. See Kevin D. O'Rourke, O.P., "Developing a Strong Catholic Identity," *Hospital Progress*, 57, n. 7 (July 1976), 88-90.

15. The text reads:

3. Insofar as the management of Catholic hospitals is concerned: a) Any cooperation which involves the approval or consent of the hospitals to actions which are in themselves, that is, by their nature and condition, directed to a contraceptive end, namely, in order that the natural effects of sexual actions deliberately performed by the sterilized subject be impeded, is absolutely forbidden. For the official approbation of direct sterilization and, *a fortiori*, its management and execution in accord with hospital regulations, is a matter which, in the objective order, is by its very nature (or intrinsically) evil. The Catholic hospital cannot cooperate with this for any reason. Any cooperation so supplied is totally unbecoming the

mission entrusted to this type of institution and would be contrary to the necessary proclamation and defense of the moral order.

b) The traditional doctrine regarding material cooperation, with the proper distinctions between necessary and free, proximate and remote, remains valid, to be applied with utmost prudence, if the case warrants.

c) In the application of the principle of material cooperation, if the case warrants, great care must be taken against scandal and the danger of any misunderstanding by an appropriate explanation of what is really being done. (*Origins*, p. 35.)

16. On cooperation, see St. Alphonsus Ligouri, *Theologia moralis*, ed. by M. Heilig (Michlin: Hanicq, 1852), II, pp. 178-89; J.P. Gury, S.J., *Compendium theologiae moralis*, 8th ed. by A. Ballerini, S.J. (Rome: Propagation Press, 1884), I, pp. 216-25; Bernard Haring, C.SS.R., *The Law of Christ*, trans. by E. G. Kaiser, C.P.P.S. (Westminster: Newman, 1961), I, pp. 292-94; Edwin Healy, S.J., *Moral Guidance* (Chicago: Loyola University Press, 1943), pp. 43-47; Gerald Kelly, S.J., *Medico-Moral Problems* (St. Louis: Catholic Hospital Association, 1954), pt. III, pp. 33-35; Augustinus Lehmkuhl, S.J., *Theologia moralis*, 10th ed. (Freiburg: Herder, 1902), I, pp. 386-407; Odon Lottin, O.S.B., *Morale fondamentale*, Biblioteque de théologie, series II, n. 1 (Paris: Desclée, 1954), pp. 289-90; J. Mausbach, *Katholische Moraltheologie*, 9th ed. by G. Ermecke (Münster: Aschendorf, 1959), I, pp. 356-62; H. Noldin, S.J., *Summa theologiae moralis*, 17th ed. by A. Schmitt, S.J. (Innsbruck: Rauch, 1941), II, pp. 117-30; M. Zalba, S.J., *Theologiae moralis summa* (Madrid: BAC, 1952), I, pp. 216-220. Charles E. Curran, "Cooperation: Toward a Revision of the Concept and Its Application," *Linacre Quarterly*, 41 (1974), 152-67. For a critique of the underlying principle of double effect, see Cornelius J. van der Poel, "The Principle of Double Effect," in *Absolutes in Moral Theology*, ed. by Charles E. Curran (Washington: Corpus Books, 1968), pp. 186-210.

17. *Summa theologica*, I, II, 18, 8, in corp.

18. See, e.g., *Taylor vs. St. Vincent's Hospital* (Billings, Montana). Although the procedure was performed in compliance with a temporary injunction, when the case came to trial the order was vacated, since in the interval Congress had passed and President Nixon signed a bill depriving the federal courts of jurisdiction (PL 93-45). The district court found the bill and its "Church amendment" constitutional. The U. S. Supreme Court refused certiorari on appeal. See *Hospital Progress*, 57, n. 4 (April, 1976), 22.

19. See *Problems in Hospital Law*, 2nd ed. (Rockville, Md.: Health Law Center, 1974).

20. Thus Zalba, *Theologia moralis*, p. 219.

21. See Harry G. Henn, *Handbook of the Law of Corporations and*

Other Business Enterprises, 2nd ed., Hornbook Series (St. Paul: West Publishing Co., 1970), pp. 352-57.

22. See, e.g., J. Y. Calvez and J. Perrin, *The Church and Social Justice*, trans. by J. R. Kirwan (Chicago: Regnery, 1961) and John F. Cronin, S.S., *Social Principles and Economic Life* (Milwaukee: Bruce, 1959).

23. On the investment policies especially of universities and churches, see, J. G. Simon, C. W. Powers and J. P. Gunnemann, *The Ethical Investor: Universities and Corporate Responsibility* (New Haven: Yale, 1972); Charles W. Powers, *Social Responsibility and Investments* (Nashville: Abingdon, 1971); *People/Profits: The Ethics of Investment* (New York: Council on Religion and International Affairs, 1972). On the multinational corporation see *The Multinational Corporation and Social Policy*, ed. by Richard A. Jackson (New York: Praeger, 1974); *The Nation-State and Transnational Corporations in Conflict: With Special Reference to Latin America*, ed. by Jon P. Gunnemann (New York: Praeger, 1975).

24. See note 15.

25. See "Suggested Medico-Moral Guidelines" for St. Michael's Hospital and St. Joseph's Hospital, Toronto, Ontario, Canada, adopted in 1974. See chapter one, pp. 22-24.

26. Such is the case with the "Policy Manual for the Committee to Advise on Requests for Obstetrical/Gynaecological Sterilization Procedures" from St. Joseph's Hospital, London, Ontario, Canada. The policy there relies on the principle of totality and has been widely imitated in the U. S.

Conclusion

Sterilization is paradigmatic of many problems facing the Church today, especially in the field of medical ethics and the Church's relationship to society. In chapter one we saw that within the past century the expansion of medical knowledge and techniques has made possible procedures that were simply not available less than a century ago. When advances in medicine made sterilization of both male and female practicable, the Church evaluated the new possibility in terms of its traditional teaching on contraception—and forbade "direct" sterilization.

The questions that have been raised about the Church's teaching on contraception have inevitably spilled over to the related issue of sterilization. The controversy has stimulated a series of investigations into the very foundations of Christian morals reviewed in chapter two. Theologians are asking again what it is that qualifies an act as morally right or wrong. They ask what grounds the moral rules that play so large a part in everyday moral decisions, and they ask just what is the appropriate role of such rules. As historical studies are done, principles long familiar in Catholic moral theology are investigated and rethought: the principle of double effect and the related principles governing cooperation have been mentioned in this study. Familiar terms like "intrinsic evil" or "direct" and "indirect" effects are the subject of continuing investigation and fresh definition. The result has been the rethinking not just of a position on a particular moral question, but of the very basis of the moral-theological enterprise itself. And a further result has been the growing gap between positions taken in statements of Church officials on a variety of moral questions, including contraception and sterilization, and the view of much of the theological community.

The rise of dissenting voices has led to study of the teaching authority of the Church: what the term means, how such teaching should be done and by whom? And there is the difficult question of the authority of statements on moral matters made by the pope, the Roman congregations and the bishops. Increasing dissatisfaction has been voiced with the highly juridical notion of *magisterium* that has dominated the Church in the nineteenth and twentieth centuries and which has asserted the exclusive right of the pope and the bishops to teach. Such a view of the *magisterium* is tied not only to a particular view of the theology of the Church, but to a particular theology of revelation and tradition as well. These theological underpinnings today seem hardly adequate to sustain an exclusively hierarchical *magisterium*. But that is not to deny the vital role of the college of bishops with the pope at its head in preserving the unity and peace of the Church, in matters of doctrine among other things. It has led, however, to a tendency to regard official Church statements as more tentative, more provisional than could have been the case with the reigning juridical model. Chapter three reviewed these new tendencies.

Developments in dogmatics and in moral theology converge when the stance of the Church-sponsored hospital with regard to sterilization is discussed. I have sketched in chapter four the factors in a vertical, rather bureaucratic model of the relationship between the hospital and Church officials and tried to suggest its inadequacies. But if the identity of Church-sponsored hospitals is not to be grounded in a juridical relationship to other Church organizations and their officers, then the urgent task of defining the role of meanings and values found in the Church's theology in giving a *raison d'être* to the hospital precisely as a religious institution comes to the fore. The hospital gives witness and, in some sense at least, teaches by the very service it gives to those who are sick. I have drawn upon Pellegrino's view of the theology of Church, of man and of sickness that must inform an authentically Catholic hospital in giving that witness.

It seems to me that the task of defining the *raison d'être* of health-care facilities sponsored by the Church is the most crucial issue that confronts them today. As federal and state legislation intervenes more and more in the planning of these facilities, it is crystal clear that institutions that are unable to explain and justify their own existence will not endure.

In this perspective the question of sterilization diminishes in importance, because it does not seem possible to me to judge sterilization a threat to the very existence of a Catholic hospital as a religiously sponsored institution. That is why cooperation in the procedure seems to me justifiable, while cooperation in abortion is not.

Of course the hospitals must continue to have guidance on difficult ethical matters from those in the Church who by their office or their professional expertise can articulate the judgment of Christian beliefs and values on a particular issue. But in weighing the goods and evils of a moral problem, the hospitals must consider the social implications of their policies too. A hospital that does not know when its commitments to Christian values demand a firm No to certain practices, like abortion on demand or the violation of the dignity of dying persons by their isolation in units where the demands of technology take precedence over human caring, has failed to consider the implications of its value commitments for its own functioning. It is, in effect, denying its very reason for existence by failing to witness to the values that it claims to uphold. Such an institution will quickly become indistinguishable from secular health-care facilities, and it is difficult to see a future for it. Loss of control over its own ethical policies and consequent loss of identity are real threats to the Catholic hospital today. The discussion of sterilization thus brings forward issues with implications for other problem areas.

Moreover, it does not seem to be too much to ask whether the meanings and values inherent in the Christian faith can continue to be institutionalized in the face of pluralism of values held by persons in the society the institutions must serve. The problem is aggravated by the increasing dependence of private health-care institutions on government funds for their construction and operation. If there is to be a future for the private, religiously sponsored hospital, the hospital must know what it is for and the implications of its commitments for patient care. I do not believe that sterilization is the issue on which the religious identity of Catholic hospitals will stand or fall. The hospitals' handling of abortion may be such an issue. In any event, I do not believe that the future of the hospitals has been predetermined. They must now find the courage to make institutional, corporate judgments on such issues as sterilization and go on to articulate their reason for existence. Only then can they survive.

INDEX

101